THE NEW PHARMACOTHERAPY OF SCHIZOPHRENIA

Clinical Practice

Number 36

Judith H. Gold, M.D., F.R.C.P.C.
Elissa P. Benedek, M.D.
Series Editors

THE NEW PHARMACOTHERAPY OF SCHIZOPHRENIA

Edited by

Alan Breier, M.D.

American Psychiatric Press, Inc.

Washington, DC
London, England

Note: The authors have worked to ensure that all information in this book concerning drug dosages, schedules, and routes of administration is accurate as of the time of publication and consistent with standards set by the U.S. Food and Drug Administration and the general medical community. As medical research and practice advance, however, therapeutic standards may change. For this reason and because human and mechanical errors sometimes occur, we recommend that readers follow the advice of a physician who is directly involved in their care or the care of a member of their family.

Manufactured in the United States of America on acid-free paper
First Edition 99 98 97 96 4 3 2 1

American Psychiatric Press, Inc.
1400 K Street, N.W., Washington, DC 20005

Library of Congress Cataloging-in-Publication Data
The new pharmacotherapy of schizophrenia / edited by Alan Breier. —
1st ed.
p. cm. — (Clinical practice series ; 36)
Includes bibliographical references and index.
ISBN 0-88048-491-8
1. Schizophrenia—Chemotherapy. 2. Antipsychotic drugs.
I. Breier, Alan, 1953– . II. Series: Clinical practice series ;
no. 36.
[DNLM: 1. Schizophrenia—drug therapy. W1 CL767J no.36 1996 / WM 203 N531555 1996]
RC514.N49 1996
616.89'82061—dc20
DNLM/DLC
for Library of Congress 95-21299
CIP

British Library Cataloguing in Publication Data
A CIP record is available from the British Library.

Contents

Contributors vii

Introduction to the Clinical Practice Series xi
Judith H. Gold, M.D., F.R.C.P.C.

Foreword xvii
William T. Carpenter, Jr., M.D.

Introduction and Overview xix
Alan Breier, M.D.

1 Clozapine: Current Status and Clinical Applications 1
Alan Breier, M.D.
Robert W. Buchanan, M.D.

2 Risperidone: Clinical Applications 15
Donna Ames, M.D.
Stephen R. Marder, M.D.
William C. Wirshing, M.D.

3 Future Antipsychotic Agents: Clinical Implications 41
Anil K. Malhotra, M.D.
Debra A. Pinsky, M.D.
Alan Breier, M.D.

4 New Neuroleptics and Experimental Antipsychotics: Future Roles 57
Adrienne C. Lahti, M.D.
Robert A. Lahti, Ph.D.
Carol A. Tamminga, M.D.

5 Conventional Neuroleptic Treatment: Current Status, Future Role 89
John M. Kane, M.D.

6 Augmenting Antipsychotic Efficacy: New Approaches 105
Laurence P. Karper, M.D.
John H. Krystal, M.D.

7 Noradrenergic Systems: A Target for Augmenting Pharmacotherapy 133
Robert E. Litman, M.D.
David Pickar, M.D.

8 Benzodiazepines 153
Owen M. Wolkowitz, M.D.

9 Treating Negative Symptoms: Pharmacological Strategies 179
Robert W. Buchanan, M.D.
Martin Brandes, M.D.
Alan Breier, M.D.

10 Treatment of Depression in Patients With Schizophrenia 205
Samuel G. Siris, M.D.

Conclusion 223
Alan Breier, M.D.

Index 225

Contributors

Donna Ames, M.D.
Staff Physician, Department of Psychiatry, West Los Angeles VA Medical Center; and Assistant Professor in Residence, Department of Psychiatry, University of California, Los Angeles, School of Medicine, Los Angeles, California

Martin Brandes, M.D.
Clinical Research Fellow, Department of Psychiatry, Maryland Psychiatric Research Center, University of Maryland School of Medicine, Baltimore, Maryland

Alan Breier, M.D.
Chief, Unit on Pathophysiology and Treatment, Experimental Therapeutics Branch, National Institutes of Health, National Institute of Mental Health, Bethesda, Maryland

Robert W. Buchanan, M.D.
Research Associate, Professor of Psychiatry, Department of Psychiatry, Maryland Psychiatric Research Center, University of Maryland School of Medicine, Baltimore, Maryland

William T. Carpenter, Jr., M.D.
Professor of Psychiatry, University of Maryland School of Medicine; and Director, Maryland Psychiatric Research Center, Baltimore, Maryland

John M. Kane, M.D.
Chairman, Department of Psychiatry, Hillside Hospital, Division of Long Island Jewish Medical Center, The Long Island Campus for the Albert Einstein College of Medicine, Glen Oaks, New York; and Professor of Psychiatry, Albert Einstein College of Medicine, Bronx, New York

Laurence P. Karper, M.D.
Assistant Professor of Psychiatry, Yale University School of Medicine; Clinical Director, Neuropsychiatric Studies Unit; and Director, Tardive Dyskinesia/Movement Disorders Clinic, West Haven VA Medical Center, West Haven, Connecticut

John H. Krystal, M.D.
Associate Professor of Psychiatry, Yale University School of Medicine; and Deputy Chief for Research and Academic Affairs, Psychiatry Service, West Haven VA Medical Center, West Haven, Connecticut

Adrienne C. Lahti, M.D.
Assistant Professor of Psychiatry, Maryland Psychiatric Research Center, University of Maryland School of Medicine, Baltimore, Maryland

Robert A. Lahti, Ph.D.
Professor of Psychiatry, Maryland Psychiatric Research Center, University of Maryland School of Medicine, Baltimore, Maryland

Robert E. Litman, M.D.
Senior Staff Fellow, Experimental Therapeutics Branch, National Institutes of Health, National Institute of Mental Health, Bethesda, Maryland

Anil K. Malhotra, M.D.
Staff Fellow, Experimental Therapeutics Branch, National Institutes of Health, National Institute of Mental Health, Bethesda, Maryland

Stephen R. Marder, M.D.
Professor of Psychiatry, Department of Psychiatry, West Los Angeles VA Medical Center and University of California, Los Angeles, School of Medicine, Los Angeles, California

David Pickar, M.D.
Chief, Experimental Therapeutics Branch, National Institutes of Health, National Institute of Mental Health, Bethesda, Maryland

Debra A. Pinsky, M.D.
Staff Fellow, Experimental Therapeutics Branch, National Institutes of Health, National Institute of Mental Health, Bethesda, Maryland

Samuel G. Siris, M.D.
Professor of Psychiatry; Director, Adult Psychiatric Day Programs, Hillside Hospital, Division of Long Island Jewish Medical Center, The Long Island Campus for the Albert Einstein College of Medicine, Glen Oaks, New York

Carol A. Tamminga, M.D.
Professor of Psychiatry and Chief, Inpatient Program, Maryland Psychiatric Research Center, University of Maryland School of Medicine, Baltimore, Maryland

William C. Wirshing, M.D.
Staff Physician, Department of Psychiatry, West Los Angeles VA Medical Center; and Associate Professor of Psychiatry, Department of Psychiatry, University of California, Los Angeles, School of Medicine, Los Angeles, California

Owen M. Wolkowitz, M.D.
Associate Professor of Psychiatry, University of California, San Francisco School of Medicine, San Francisco, California

Introduction
to the Clinical Practice Series

Over the years of its existence the series of monographs entitled *Clinical Insights* gradually became focused on providing current, factual, and theoretical material of interest to the clinician working outside of a hospital setting. To reflect this orientation, the name of the Series has been changed to *Clinical Practice.*

The Clinical Practice Series will provide books that give the mental health clinician a practical, clinical approach to a variety of psychiatric problems. These books will provide up-to-date literature reviews and emphasize the most recent treatment methods. Thus, the publications in the Series will interest clinicians working both in psychiatry and in the other mental health professions.

Each year a number of books will be published dealing with all aspects of clinical practice. In addition, from time to time when appropriate, the publications may be revised and updated. Thus, the Series will provide quick access to relevant and important areas of psychiatric practice. Some books in the Series will be authored by a person considered to be an expert in that particular area; others will be edited by such an expert, who will also draw together other knowledgeable authors to produce a comprehensive overview of that topic.

Some of the books in the Clinical Practice Series will have their foundation in presentations at an annual meeting of the American Psychiatric Association. All will contain the most recently available information on the subjects discussed. Theoretical and scientific data will be applied to clinical situations, and case illustrations will be utilized in order to make the material even more relevant for the practitioner. Thus, the Clinical Practice Series should provide educational reading in a compact format especially designed for the mental health clinician–psychiatrist.

Judith H. Gold, M.D., F.R.C.P.C.
Series Editor
Clinical Practice Series

Clinical Practice Series Titles

The New Pharmacotherapy of Schizophrenia (#36)
Edited by Alan Breier, M.D.

Clinical Assessment and Management of Severe Personality Disorders (#35)
Edited by Paul S. Links, M.D., M.Sc., F.R.C.P.C.

Predictors of Treatment Response in Mood Disorders (#34)
Edited by Paul J. Goodnick, M.D.

Successful Psychiatric Practice: Current Dilemmas, Choices, and Solutions (#33)
Edited by Edward K. Silberman, M.D.

Alternatives to the Hospital for Acute Psychiatric Treatment (#32)
Edited by Richard Warner, M.B., D.P.M.

Behavioral Complications in Alzheimer's Disease (#31)
Edited by Brian A. Lawlor, M.D.

Patient Violence and the Clinician (#30)
Edited by Burr S. Eichelman, M.D., Ph.D., and Anne C. Hartwig, J.D., Ph.D.

Effective Use of Group Therapy in Managed Care (#29)
Edited by K. Roy MacKenzie, M.D., F.R.C.P.C.

Rediscovering Childhood Trauma: Historical Casebook and Clinical Applications (#28)
Edited by Jean M. Goodwin, M.D., M.P.H.

Treatment of Adult Survivors of Incest (#27)
Edited by Patricia L. Paddison, M.D.

Madness and Loss of Motherhood: Sexuality, Reproduction, and Long-Term Mental Illness (#26)
Edited by Roberta J. Apfel, M.D., M.P.H., and Maryellen H. Handel, Ph.D.

Psychiatric Aspects of Symptom Management in Cancer Patients (#25)
Edited by William Breitbart, M.D., and Jimmie C. Holland, M.D.

Responding to Disaster: A Guide for Mental Health Professionals (#24)
Edited by Linda S. Austin, M.D.

Psychopharmacological Treatment Complications in the Elderly (#23)
Edited by Charles A. Shamoian, M.D., Ph.D.

Anxiety Disorders in Children and Adolescents (#22)
By Syed Arshad Husain, M.D., F.R.C.P.C., F.R.C.Psych., and Javad Kashani, M.D.

Suicide and Clinical Practice (#21)
Edited by Douglas Jacobs, M.D.

Special Problems in Managing Eating Disorders (#20)
Edited by Joel Yager, M.D., Harry E. Gwirtsman, M.D., and Carole K. Edelstein, M.D.

Children and AIDS (#19)
Edited by Margaret L. Stuber, M.D.

Current Treatments of Obsessive-Compulsive Disorder (#18)
Edited by Michele Tortora Pato, M.D., and Joseph Zohar, M.D.

Benzodiazepines in Clinical Practice: Risks and Benefits (#17)
Edited by Peter P. Roy-Byrne, M.D., and Deborah S. Cowley, M.D.

Adolescent Psychotherapy (#16)
Edited by Marcia Slomowitz, M.D.

Family Approaches in Treatment of Eating Disorders (#15)
Edited by D. Blake Woodside, M.D., M.Sc., F.R.C.P.C., and Lorie Shekter-Wolfson, M.S.W., C.S.W.

Clinical Management of Gender Identity Disorders in Children and Adults (#14)
Edited by Ray Blanchard, Ph.D., and Betty W. Steiner, M.B., F.R.C.P.C.

New Perspectives on Narcissism (#13)
Edited by Eric M. Plakun, M.D.

The Psychosocial Impact of Job Loss (#12)
By Nick Kates, M.B.B.S., F.R.C.P.C., Barrie S. Greiff, M.D., and Duane Q. Hagen, M.D.

Office Treatment of Schizophrenia (#11)
Edited by Mary V. Seeman, M.D., F.R.C.P.C., and Stanley E. Greben, M.D., F.R.C.P.C.

Psychiatric Care of Migrants: A Clinical Guide (#10)
By Joseph Westermeyer, M.D., M.P.H., Ph.D.

Family Involvement in Treatment of the Frail Elderly (#9)
Edited by Marion Zucker Goldstein, M.D.

Measuring Mental Illness: Psychometric Assessment for Clinicians (#8)
Edited by Scott Wetzler, Ph.D.

Juvenile Homicide (#7)
Edited by Elissa P. Benedek, M.D., and Dewey G. Cornell, Ph.D.

The Neuroleptic Malignant Syndrome and Related Conditions (#6)
By Arthur Lazarus, M.D., Stephan C. Mann, M.D., and Stanley N. Caroff, M.D.

Anxiety: New Findings for the Clinician (#5)
Edited by Peter Roy-Byrne, M.D.

Anxiety and Depressive Disorders in the Medical Patient (#4)
By Leonard R. Derogatis, Ph.D., and Thomas N. Wise, M.D.

Family Violence: Emerging Issues of a National Crisis (#3)
Edited by Leah J. Dickstein, M.D., and Carol C. Nadelson, M.D.

Divorce as a Developmental Process (#2)
Edited by Judith H. Gold, M.D., F.R.C.P.C.

Treating Chronically Mentally Ill Women (#1)
Edited by Leona L. Bachrach, Ph.D., and Carol C. Nadelson, M.D.

Foreword

Schizophrenia is highly personal in its devastating effects on intimacy, rapport, volition, affect, cognition, perception, and the capacity for gratification. From the observer's perspective, schizophrenia creates bizarre behavior, perception without stimulus, peculiar interpretation of the ordinary, and the tearing asunder of shared experience. The social cost is high, ranging from personal neglect and homelessness to extensive clinical care and loss of productivity. The financial burden of this disease exceeds that of cancer in the United States. Given the scope of the problem, funding the acquisition of new knowledge through science is astoundingly low, a societal neglect attributable to the effects of stigma on a poorly informed public.

No prevention or cure exists for schizophrenia, but extremely important therapeutic advances have prepared the field for a most exciting future. The clinician can rely on increasingly critical scientific evaluation of new treatments. Several psychosocial therapeutic approaches have been recently found efficacious in randomized, controlled trials, and the neuroscience community is discovering schizophrenia while the pharmaceutical industry rediscovers this illness.

This new era of schizophrenia therapeutics is being introduced with many candidate drugs, a range of hypothesized therapeutic actions going far beyond dopamine receptor blockade, and treatment effects intended to address pathological and functional attributes of schizophrenia well beyond psychotic symptom reduction and relapse prevention.

Alan Breier, M.D., has brought together the clinical leaders of this new generation of schizophrenia therapeutics, and they provide a comprehensive, critical, and very readable analysis of current advances. Physician and nonphysician clinicians will find this a trustworthy guide for clinical application of the recently introduced antipsychotic drugs and a critical reassessment of the present and future role of conventional neuroleptic drugs. Special attention is given to the treatment of negative symptoms and depression. Pharmacological strategies targeting noradrenergic, γ-aminobutyric acid (GABA)ergic, serotonergic, and dopamine agonistic properties with available drugs are presented, providing the clinician with new approaches for enhancing antipsychotic effects.

This book presents cutting-edge information that should remarkably alter current approaches to treatment. In addition, the reader is treated to a view of future development of experimental drugs and an overview that provides perspective and integration for this rapidly developing area of clinical science.

William T. Carpenter, Jr., M.D.

Introduction and Overview

Alan Breier, M.D.

Schizophrenia is the most severe psychiatric disorder and, as noted in an editorial in *Nature,* it is "arguably the worst disease affecting mankind, even AIDS not excepted" (1988, pp. 95–96). The public health facts support this claim. Schizophrenia is a common illness affecting approximately 1% of the population, or 2.6 million United States citizens. The illness is debilitating and usually chronic, as demonstrated by the fact that patients with schizophrenia occupy 25% of all hospital beds and account for 40% of all long-term-care days (Talbott et al. 1987). The costs associated with lost productivity and treatment are approximately $30 billion annually (Rupp and Keith 1993). Excessive mortality is associated with this illness, with a 20% shorter life expectancy compared with the general population and a 10% suicide rate (Breier and Astrachan 1984). It may be concluded that schizophrenia represents a public health crisis for the nation, which calls for urgent progress in the treatment of this illness.

The first era in the modern pharmacotherapy of this illness began in the early 1950s with the serendipitous discovery followed by confirmation that chlorpromazine was an effective antipsychotic agent. Chlorpromazine and the subsequent neuroleptics offered unequivocal clinical improvement for the majority of patients with schizophrenia, and their worldwide utilization dramatically changed the clinical landscape of this illness. However, neuroleptic drugs rarely result in complete symptom remission and return to premorbid levels of functioning. In fact, a substantial number of patients with schizophrenia derive little or no benefit from these drugs. Moreover, their side effects, such as extrapyramidal symptoms and tardive dyskinesia, contribute to personal discomfort, noncompliance, physical disfigurement, and disability. It may be argued that since the introduction of chlorpromazine 40 years ago, there has been no significant breakthrough in the pharmacotherapy of schizophrenia until recently.

The premise of this volume is that we are at the threshold of a new era in the pharmacotherapy of schizophrenia. This second era is characterized by a new class of antipsychotic agents that promises superior efficacy and more favorable side-effect profiles and by an improved understanding of how to use existing pharmacotherapeutic agents. It may well be that 5–10 years from now, a whole new class of pharmacotherapeutic agents will replace the traditional neuroleptics as the mainstay for treating this illness.

The drug most responsible for this new pharmacotherapeutic era is clozapine. The first chapter assesses its current status and clinical applications. Chapter 2 focuses on risperidone, which is becoming a widely used first-line antipsychotic agent. Chapters 3 and 4 explore clinical aspects and mechanisms of action of new and experimental antipsychotic agents. In Chapter 5, the author reviews the current status of the traditional neuroleptic agents, and Chapters 6 and 7 examine approaches to augmenting traditional neuroleptic drug efficacy through the use of "add-on" agents. Chapter 8 reviews the role of benzodiazepines in the treatment of schizophrenia. The two remaining chapters focus on treatment strategies developed specifically for two common and debilitating symptom clusters of schizophrenia—negative symptoms and depression. A primary goal of this volume is to equip both the clinician and researcher with new information for the improved treatment of this severe and complicated illness.

References

Editorial. Nature 336:95–96, 1988

Breier A, Astrachan BM: Characterization of schizophrenic patients who commit suicide. Am J Psychiatry 141:206–209, 1984

Rupp A, Keith SJ: The costs of schizophrenia: assessing the burden. Psychiatr Clin North Am 16:413–423, 1993

Talbott JA, Goldman HH, Ross L: Schizophrenia: an economic perspective. Psychiatric Annals 17:577–579, 1987

CHAPTER 1

Clozapine: Current Status and Clinical Applications

Alan Breier, M.D.
Robert W. Buchanan, M.D.

The modern era of the pharmacotherapy of schizophrenia began in the early 1950s when chlorpromazine was found to be an effective antipsychotic agent for patients with schizophrenia. Chlorpromazine was the first effective pharmacological treatment for this illness and served as a reference or model for the development of subsequent antipsychotic agents. These "Thorazine-like" drugs are known as neuroleptics because, in addition to antipsychotic efficacy, they produce neurological side effects known as extrapyramidal side effects (EPS).

Neuroleptic drugs have had an enormous effect on the clinical management of schizophrenia and other psychotic illnesses. One example is the paradigm shift from long-term residential care in state hospitals before the 1950s to community-based outpatient care. The extent of deinstitutionalism seen today would not have been possible without the neuroleptic drugs.

Although neuroleptics are unequivocally superior to placebo for schizophrenia (see Chapter 5 in this volume), they are far from ideal treatments. Estimates suggest that 15% of patients with schizophrenia are essentially resistant to the therapeutic effects of neuroleptics. This group of patients is known as *treatment resistant*. Approximately 70% of all patients with schizophrenia derive benefit from neuroleptics but still have clinically apparent positive (e.g., hallucinations, delusions, formal thought disorder) and/or negative (e.g., lack of social drive, constricted affect) symptoms and functional deficits. This group of patients is known as *partial responders.* Only approximately 15% of patients with schizophrenia derive "optimal" symptom control and restoration of functional status. Thus, 85% of patients are gleaning suboptimal responses from traditional neuroleptics. These data, coupled with the fact that neuroleptics cause EPS and are associated with a 4%–5% per year incidence of tardive dyskinesia, indicate that the traditional neuroleptics are not adequate for the treatment of schizophrenia.

Since the discovery of chlorpromazine's antipsychotic efficacy nearly 40 years ago, many drugs have been developed for the treatment of schizophrenia, with the hope that they would have superior efficacy to chlorpromazine. However, since the early 1950s, not one agent has fulfilled this hope. The first agent to demonstrate superiority to traditional neuroleptic drugs is clozapine.

History of Clozapine

Clozapine is not a new drug; it was developed in the 1960s. In the early 1970s, clinical trials established that clozapine was an effective antipsychotic drug. Further trials suggested that clozapine had a favorable clinical profile with no EPS. In 1975, 13 clozapine-treated patients in Finland developed agranulocytosis, which resulted in eight deaths (Griffith and Saameli 1975). As would be expected, interest in clozapine dramatically dropped, and a plan to eliminate clozapine was proposed by Sandoz, the pharmaceutical company that produces clozapine. However, because of a relatively small number of psychiatrists and patients' family members who indicated that certain clozapine-treated patients were deriving symptom control that was far superior to what was achieved with previous antipsychotic drugs, clozapine was made available on a limited, compassionate-need basis for the most severely ill patients.

For the next 10 years, the use of clozapine slowly increased, particularly in Europe. The reports from Europe supported earlier claims that clozapine appeared to have superior efficacy compared with traditional neuroleptics in treatment-resistant patients with schizophrenia and did not produce EPS. The rate of clozapine-induced agranulocytosis was determined to be approximately 1%–2%, and cessation of clozapine resulted in return of the white blood cell (WBC) count to normal levels. In part because no promising alternative treatments were available for severely treatment-resistant patients with schizophrenia and because of the desperate plight of these patients, a multicenter trial of clozapine in the most severely ill, neuroleptic treatment–resistant patients with schizophrenia was conducted in the United States. This study was known as Study 30.

Multicenter Trial of Clozapine in Treatment-Resistant Schizophrenia: Study 30

John Kane, Herbert Meltzer, and Gilbert Honigfeld were principally responsible for the design, implementation, and data analysis/reporting of Study 30 (Kane et al. 1988). Sixteen inpatient treatment centers across the United States participated in the study and collectively enrolled 268 patients with a diagnosis of schizophrenia. Patients fulfilled rigorous a priori criteria for neuroleptic treatment resistance, which included failure to improve after trials of at least three different traditional neuroleptic drugs and then a prospective, 6-week trial of haloperidol (mean ± SD daily dose: 61 ± 4 mg/day). The patients in this sample were noteworthy in terms of their chronicity, with a duration of current hospitalization of 216 ± 321 weeks, and they had 9.2 ± 7 previous hospitalizations. Following the prospective haloperidol trial, patients were randomized to a double-blind, 6-week trial of either clozapine (up to 900 mg/day) or chlorpromazine (up to 1,800 mg/day).

The extraordinary results of this study were published in 1988 (Kane et al. 1988). Clozapine demonstrated superiority to chlorpromazine for Brief Psychiatric Rating Scale (BPRS; Overall and Gorham 1962) positive and negative symptoms. Significant differences occurred for positive symptoms after only 1 week of treatment and for negative symptoms after only 2 weeks of treatment. Moreover, clozapine was superior for measures of functioning and global symptomatology. Thirty percent of clozapine-treated patients and only 4% of chlorpromazine-treated patients fulfilled a priori responder criteria. Thus, this was the first study that conclusively demonstrated that an agent had clinical superiority to traditional neuroleptics, and these results paved the way for Food and Drug Administration (FDA) approval of clozapine in the United States.

Indications for Clozapine

One of the most important clinical questions that emerged from the multicenter clozapine trial was "Who should receive clozapine?" The multicenter data confirmed that clozapine had superior efficacy in the most severely ill, treatment-refractory inpatients with schizophrenia, but it was unknown whether this efficacy profile would generalize to less ill patients with schizophrenia and other patient groups. Since the 1990 FDA approval of clozapine for treatment-resistant schizophrenia, neuroleptic intolerance, and severe tardive dyskinesia, a number of studies that were initiated are providing data that suggest that a much broader application of this agent may be indicated.

Chronic Outpatient Schizophrenia

Because the largest subgroup of patients with schizophrenia are outpatients and conventional neuroleptics do not eliminate positive and negative symptoms and do not result in return to premorbid levels of functioning for the majority of these patients, we conducted a study to assess clozapine's efficacy in chronically ill, moderately symptomatic outpatients with schizophrenia. The study design included a 6-week trial of fluphenazine to ensure stability and the presence of residual positive and/or negative symptoms, followed by randomization to either a 10-week double-blind trial of clozapine (400 mg/day) or haloperidol (20 mg/day). After the 10-week double-blind phase, clozapine-treated patients were followed for 1 year.

Data analyses revealed that clozapine was superior to haloperidol for positive symptoms and measures of hostility (Breier et al. 1994). Thus, these data indicate that clozapine has a therapeutic role in chronically ill, stable outpatients. In addition, the results to date of the 1-year outcome studies demonstrated that clozapine was effective in reducing relapses and hospitalizations (Breier et al. 1993). From a clinical perspective, we have been particularly impressed with clozapine's ability to stabilize the course of illness. In fact, we have observed a number of cases of improved stability even when significant reductions in psychotic symptoms did not occur. The significant decrease in relapses and hospitalization rates has been found by others (Meltzer et al. 1990), and Meltzer et al. (1993) have provided cost-analysis data suggesting that the decrease in relapses/hospitalizations leads to an overall cost savings with clozapine therapy when patients are treated for at least 2 years. It is important to address this issue in a carefully controlled prospective study.

In addition to its superior efficacy, we found that there were no significant obstacles to initiation of clozapine treatment on an outpatient basis, and overall the drug was well tolerated. Thus, we recommended that clozapine be considered in outpatients who have not achieved complete symptom remission with traditional neuroleptics.

Treatment-Resistant Childhood Schizophrenia

Judy Rapoport and her colleagues at the National Institute of Mental Health (NIMH) Intramural Program in Bethesda, Maryland, are conducting a double-blind study of clozapine versus haloperidol in patients with childhood schizophrenia who have not achieved symptom remission with traditional neuroleptics. Preliminary analysis suggests that outcomes are strikingly similar to those observed in previous studies of adult-onset schizophrenia. If these data hold up, clozapine would be a treatment option for this clinical population.

Treatment-Resistant Bipolar Illness

Data that are emerging from a few centers indicate that clozapine is an effective treatment for treatment-resistant bipolar illness (Suppes et al. 1992). Preliminary data from a double-blind study by Joseph Calibrese at Case-Western Reserve in Cleveland, Ohio, suggest that clozapine has both robust antimanic and antipsychotic efficacy. In fact, it appears to have more impressive effects on symptom reduction in this population than in patients with chronic schizophrenia.

Psychosis Induced by Dopaminergic Treatments in Parkinson's Disease

A problem faced by clinicians in the treatment of Parkinson's disease is psychosis induced by dopaminergic treatments. Traditional neuroleptics have marginal utility in these cases because they antagonize the therapeutic benefits of L-dopa and other dopaminergic treatments for Parkinson's disease. Very low doses of clozapine (e.g., 25–75 mg/day), however, have been shown to prevent psychosis without interfering with the therapeutic benefits of dopaminergic treatments (Wolk and Douglas 1992). The mechanism is believed to be related to the difference in dopamine D_2-receptor binding between clozapine and traditional neuroleptics. Clozapine has much lower D_2 occupancy in the basal ganglia than the traditional agents (Farde et al. 1988). The motor abnormalities of Parkinson's disease are caused by dopamine depletion in the basal ganglia. Thus, traditional neuroleptics antagonize basal ganglia dopamine replacement therapy, which undermines treatment of Parkinson's motor symptoms, whereas clozapine does not.

United States Responder Rates for Chronic Schizophrenia

Table 1–1 contains a summary of United States studies of clozapine in patients with chronic schizophrenia since and inclusive of Study 30. All of the studies used admission criteria that included a history of inadequate response to conventional neuroleptic drugs. The responder rates are based on what is considered clinically meaningful symptom reduction (usually 20% reduction in BPRS scores). As noted, there have been seven studies, with duration of clozapine treatment ranging from 6 weeks to 1 year. Responder rates ranged from 30% to 62%. Thirty percent, which was found in the multicenter study, is probably an outlier because of the short duration of treatment (i.e., 6 weeks) and the fact that there was no evidence of a plateauing of effects suggesting that a longer trial would have resulted in a higher responder rate. Thus,

Table 1–1. Clozapine responder rates in chronic schizophrenia United States studies

	N	Illness severity	Trial	Responders (%)
Kane et al. 1988	126 inpatients	++++	6 weeks	30
Meltzer et al. 1990	51 inpatients	+++	6 months	61
Conley 1992[a]	25 inpatients	++++	1 year	60
Wilson 1992	37 inpatients	++++	6 months	62
Breier et al. 1993	30 outpatients	++	1 year	60
Zito et al. 1993	152 inpatients	++++	1 year	43
Pickar et al. 1994	40 inpatients	+++	4 months	50

Note. ++ = moderate severity; +++ = very severe; ++++ = extreme severity.
[a]Personal communication.

the existing data suggest that 40%–60% of chronically ill patients with schizophrenia who are treated for a minimum of 4 months may anticipate a clinically meaningful response to clozapine.

Predictors of Clinical Improvement

As noted from the studies above, a substantial number of clozapine-treated patients do not derive clinical improvement beyond that attained with conventional neuroleptics. However, currently, no good clinical predictors identify which patients will and will not have good responses to clozapine. Several clinical variables, however, have been significantly related to a good clozapine outcome. These variables include high levels of EPS on traditional neuroleptics, later illness onset, shorter duration of illness, female gender, and paranoid subtype (Meltzer 1992; Pickar et al. 1992). Interestingly, these variables (with the exception of EPS) are among a group of characteristics that are considered good prognostic variables for schizophrenia in general. Although the relation of these variables to clozapine outcome was significant, it was not robust and failed to account for enough variance to be clinically useful for deciding who should be prescribed clozapine. More research in this area is clearly needed. Another factor that has been found to be predictive of clozapine outcome is plasma level of clozapine. Patients with plasma levels above 350 ng/ml tended to have better clozapine responses than patients with levels below 350 ng/ml (Perry et al. 1991). Clozapine dose is related to plasma level, which underscores the importance of an adequate dose during clozapine treatment.

Adequate Length of a Clozapine Trial

The question of how long to treat a patient with clozapine before deciding to terminate clozapine treatment versus committing to extended therapy is important because the risk of agranulocytosis and cost of clozapine (average cost is approximately $5,000 annually) mandate that the shortest trial possible be pursued in nonresponders. Early reports suggested that up to a full year of clozapine treatment may be needed to identify responders. We examined this issue in a 1-year outcome study and found that 95% of all responders to clozapine were identified within the first 4 months of treatment (Figure 1–1) (Breier et al. 1993). Our clinical experience is that, when an adequate dose is used, it is exceedingly rare for a patient to show no evidence of clozapine response during the first 4 months of treatment and then later improve significantly. Thus, we recommend a clozapine trial of 4–6 months as sufficient to determine whether a patient is a candidate for longer-term clozapine therapy.

Effects on Negative Symptoms

The multicenter study (Study 30) described above found that clozapine was superior to chlorpromazine for negative symptoms (i.e., anergy). This was exciting because negative symptoms are among the most debilitating features of schizophrenia, and traditional antipsychotic agents tend not to be very effective for these symptoms (see Chapter 9 in this volume). Some subsequent studies also demonstrated that clozapine appeared to be an effective treatment for negative symptoms. We examined this issue in a double-blind comparison of clozapine versus haloperidol in chronically ill outpatients described above (Breier et al. 1994). We found a significant difference between clozapine and haloperidol

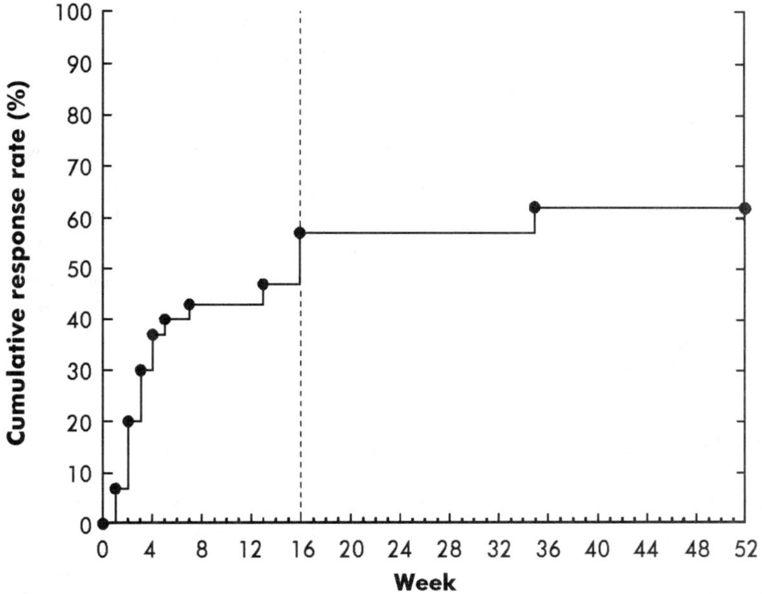

Figure 1–1. Cumulative response rates of 30 outpatients with schizophrenia during a 1-year trial of clozapine.

for negative symptoms (Scale for the Assessment of Negative Symptoms [SANS; Andreasen 1981] total score), but this was attributable to only a minor decrease in negative symptoms during clozapine treatment and a minor worsening of negative symptoms during haloperidol treatment.

One of the many aspects of our study that differed from Study 30 and other studies suggesting that clozapine has superior efficacy for negative symptoms is levels of preexisting (baseline) EPS. Outpatients in our study had very low levels of EPS, whereas outpatients in the other studies had moderate to high EPS levels. It is clearly established that clozapine does not produce EPS, and preexisting levels of EPS significantly decrease during clozapine treatment. It is also clear that EPS may mimic negative symptoms. Thus, we hypothesized that previous reports of clozapine's effects on negative symptoms may be an epiphenomenon that is driven by clozapine's lack of EPS-inducing effects. To pursue this issue further, we examined the effects of clozapine versus haloperidol in a subgroup of patients who had primary negative symptoms (i.e., negative symptoms that were not secondary to EPS or other possible causes of negative symptoms such as depression and psychosis). We found that in this group, negative symptom levels did not change (Breier et al. 1994). Based on these data, we predict that clozapine may reduce secondary negative symptoms in patients with schizophrenia when the primary source of the negative symptoms (i.e., EPS, depression, psychosis) is improved; however, clozapine will not reduce primary enduring negative symptoms. Clearly, the issue of clozapine's effects on negative symptoms is far from resolved.

Incidence and Predictors of Agranulocytosis

In a study of 11,555 patients receiving clozapine and participating in a weekly WBC monitoring program from February 1990 to April 1991, Alvir and colleagues (1993) examined the incidence and risk factors associated with clozapine-induced agranulocytosis. Of the 11,555 patients, 73 developed agranulocytosis. The cumulative incidence of agranulocytosis was 0.80% at 1 year and 0.91% at 1.5 years. Of the 73 patients who developed agranulocytosis, 70 cases occurred in the first 6 months of clozapine therapy. Thus, the risk of agranulocytosis is dramatically reduced after the first 6 months of treatment. In fact, several European countries do not require weekly WBC monitoring after the first 4–6 months of clozapine therapy. Two patients who developed agranulocytosis died of sepsis, which underlines the fact that even though the risk of death is quite low, it may occur; therefore, a high level of diligence is necessary among clinicians prescribing clozapine. In all other patients, WBC counts returned to normal after clozapine was discontinued. Studies are under way to examine methods to hasten the return to normal WBC counts with granulocyte colony-stimulating factor (Oren et al. 1993), which may lower the risk of complications secondary to clozapine-induced agranulocytosis.

The risk of agranulocytosis increases with age, which suggests that extra caution is necessary when clozapine is given to elderly patients (Alvir et al. 1993). In addition, women are at higher risk for agranulocytosis (Alvir et al. 1993). The conclusion that may be drawn from the data is that agranulocytosis is a substantial hazard of clozapine administration, but this hazard can be reduced by weekly WBC monitoring.

Other Side Effects

The most common side effect of clozapine is sedation, which occurs in approximately 40% of clozapine-treated patients. Like many clozapine-related side effects (with the exception of agranulocytosis), sedation is dose dependent. It tends to occur early in treatment and can be mitigated with slow dose titrations. Other relatively common side effects are tachycardia (25%), salivation (30%), and weight gain. Tachycardia may be managed with low-dose β-blockers. Other side effects include orthostatic hypotension, dizziness, constipation, and nausea. A dose-dependent increase in the incidence of generalized seizures occurs in approximately 6%–8% of patients on doses above 600 mg/day. At low clozapine doses, the seizure incidence does not appear to be any greater than that with conventional neuroleptics. Use of valproic acid or phenytoin is recommended in conjunction with clozapine in patients who have had clozapine-induced seizures. Transient fever has been observed in about 10%–20% of patients during the initial weeks of clozapine treatment. This is generally benign and self-limiting. However, a WBC count should always be checked if fever rises. Also, neuroleptic malignant syndrome has been reported during clozapine treatment (Miller et al. 1991) and should be considered in the differential diagnosis.

Conclusion

The establishment of clozapine as a superior pharmacotherapeutic agent for chronic schizophrenia is perhaps the most significant advance in the research of this illness in decades. Clozapine has replaced chlorpromazine and haloperidol as the new reference or model for the development of future antipsychotic agents. These future agents promise to provide improved clinical efficacy and no EPS/tardive dyskinesia (see Chapter 3 in this volume). Although it has taken 40 years, clozapine is marking a new era in the pharmacotherapy of schizophrenia.

References

Alvir JMJ, Lieberman JA, Safferman AZ, et al: Clozapine-induced agranulocytosis: incidence and risk factors in the United States. N Engl J Med 329:162–167, 1993

Andreasen NC: The Scale for the Assessment of Negative Symptoms (SANS). Iowa City, IA, University of Iowa, 1981

Breier A, Buchanan RW, Irish D, et al: Clozapine treatment of outpatients with schizophrenia: outcome and long-term response patterns. Hosp Community Psychiatry 44:1145–1149, 1993

Breier A, Buchanan RW, Kirkpatrick B, et al: Effects of clozapine on positive and negative symptoms in outpatients with schizophrenia. Am J Psychiatry 151:20–26, 1994

Farde L, Wiesel F-A, Halldin C, et al: Central D_2 dopamine receptor occupancy in schizophrenic patients treated with antipsychotic drugs. Arch Gen Psychiatry 45:71–76, 1988

Griffith RW, Saameli K: Clozapine and agranulocytosis. Lancet 2:657, 1975

Kane J, Honigfeld G, Singer J, et al: Clozapine for the treatment-resistant schizophrenic: a double-blind comparison with chlorpromazine. Arch Gen Psychiatry 45:789–796, 1988

Meltzer HY: Treatment of the neuroleptic-nonresponsive schizophrenic patient. Schizophr Bull 18:515–542, 1992

Meltzer HY, Burnett S, Bastani B, et al: Effects of six months of clozapine treatment on the quality of life of chronic schizophrenic patients. Hosp Community Psychiatry 41:892–897, 1990

Meltzer HY, Cola P, Way L, et al: Cost effectiveness of clozapine in neuroleptic-resistant schizophrenia. Am J Psychiatry 150:1630–1638, 1993

Miller DD, Sharafuddin MJA, Kathol RG: A case of clozapine-induced neuroleptic malignant syndrome. J Clin Psychiatry 52:99–101, 1991

Oren R, Granat E, Shtrussberg S, et al: Clozapine-induced agranulocytosis treated with granulocyte macrophage colony stimulating factor. Br J Psychiatry 162:686–687, 1993

Overall JE, Gorham DR: The Brief Psychiatric Rating Scale. Psychol Rep 10:799–812, 1962

Perry PJ, Miller DD, Arndt SV, et al: Clozapine and norclozapine plasma concentrations and clinical response of treatment-refractory schizophrenic patients. Am J Psychiatry 148:231–235, 1991

Pickar D, Owen RR, Litman RE, et al: Clinical and biologic response to clozapine in patients with schizophrenia: crossover comparison with fluphenazine. Arch Gen Psychiatry 49:345–353, 1992

Pickar D, Owen RR, Litman RE, et al: Predictors of clozapine response in schizophrenia. J Clin Psychiatry 55 (suppl B):9, 1994

Suppes T, McElroy SL, Gilbert J, et al: Clozapine in the treatment of dysphoric mania. Biol Psychiatry 32:270–280, 1992

Wilson WH: Clinical review of clozapine treatment in a state hospital. Hosp Community Psychiatry 43:700–703, 1992

Wolk SI, Douglas CJ: Clozapine treatment of psychosis in Parkinson's disease: a report of five consecutive cases. J Clin Psychiatry 53:373–377, 1992

Zito JM, Volavka J, Craig TJ, et al: Pharmacoepidemiology of clozapine in 202 inpatients with schizophrenia. Ann Pharmacother 27:1262–1269, 1993

CHAPTER 2

Risperidone: Clinical Applications

Donna Ames, M.D.
Stephen R. Marder, M.D.
William C. Wirshing, M.D.

For almost four decades, the mainstay of psychopharmacological treatment of patients with schizophrenia has been medications that block dopamine (D_2) receptors (Seeman et al. 1976). Conventional D_2 blocking agents have several limitations. They are effective for only 70% of patients who take them. These treatment responders have high rate of noncompliance that is thought to be largely due to intolerable extrapyramidal side effects (EPS) such as akinesia and akathisia (Van Putten 1974). In addition to intolerable side effects, conventional antipsychotics are not effective in treating all symptoms of schizophrenia. Although they diminish positive symptoms of schizophrenia (auditory hallucinations and delusions), they are substantially less effective against negative symptoms (blunted affect and emotional withdrawal). There is a great need to find new antipsychotic agents that are more effective for both positive and negative symptoms and that produce less EPS. Risperidone is one of many molecules—the putative "atypical" antipsychotic medications—that has been added to our pharmacological armamentarium.

Atypical Antipsychotic Medications

Definition

By broad definition, an *atypical* antipsychotic medication exerts its effect without causing either EPS or elevations of prolactin in humans (Meltzer 1989; Meltzer et al. 1989). Many preclinical models have been used to develop potential atypical antipsychotic agents. In the rat model, antipsychotic efficacy is determined by inhibition of conditioned responses and apomorphine-induced hyperactivity. EPS liability in humans is thought to parallel the inhibition of oral stereotypies and the induction of catalepsy in rats. Atypical agents generally inhibit stereotypies and induce catalepsy at 3–10 times the dose necessary to inhibit hyperactivity.

The precise mechanism responsible for these atypical properties is unknown. Clozapine, the prototypic atypical agent, exerts its action at D_1, D_2, D_3, D_4, 5-HT_2, and 5-HT_3 receptors. Clozapine blocks serotonin receptors (5-HT_2) 10 times more potently than D_2 receptors. Positron-emission tomography (PET) scan studies demonstrate this high 5-HT_2-receptor binding affinity in humans (Farde et al. 1992). 5-HT_2 blockade reverses D_2 blockade–induced catalepsy in rats. This may explain clozapine's low EPS potential (Mizuki et al. 1990; Silver et al. 1991).

Serotonin has an inhibitory effect on mesocortical dopamine (DA) neurons. 5-HT_2 blockade results in disinhibition of these DA neurons and may lead to enhanced DA function in the frontal lobes. Hypodopaminergic function in the frontal lobes has been implicated in the production of negative symptoms. Thus, clozapine's 5-HT_2 blockade may account for its superior efficacy in the treatment of negative symptoms. Clozapine's effect on serotonin receptors prompted a search for other compounds that specifically antagonize 5-HT_2 receptors. Mianserin, cyproheptadine, and ritanserin are fairly specific 5-HT_2 blocking agents that have been tested in patients with schizophrenia. The development of ritanserin, and ultimately risperidone, has been largely a search for agents that exploit this postulated mechanism of clozapine's action.

Ritanserin and Other 5-HT_2 Blocking Agents

Ritanserin is a highly potent and reasonably specific serotonin antagonist for 5-HT_2 and 5-HT_{1c} receptors. It was originally developed as an agent to improve sleep. Jouvet, in 1969, first demonstrated that serotonin was involved in the production of slow-wave sleep in animals. Ritanserin increases slow-wave sleep in healthy humans (Declerck et al. 1987; Idzikowski et al. 1986). Abnormalities in slow-wave sleep may contribute to many neuropsychiatric disturbances, including dysthymia, anxiety disorders, and the negative symptoms of schizophrenia (Janssen 1988). Benson and colleagues (1991) examined ritanserin's effects on slow-wave sleep in schizophrenia. They found that rapid eye movement (REM) sleep was increased and fewer awakenings occurred with ritanserin treatment. They did not observe a change in slow-wave sleep. Because sleep disruption is an accepted component of depression, ritanserin might be useful as a thymosthenic agent. It reduced the symptoms in patients with dysthymia and generalized anxiety (Reyntjens et al. 1986).

Not only is serotonin important in sleep, but it also regulates movement through its antagonistic effect on DA transmission in basal ganglia structures. Electrophysiological studies in animals suggest that 5-HT_2 antagonism with ritanserin increases firing in DA neurons (Ugedo et al. 1989). Ritanserin has been used in a small trial in the treatment of parkinsonian tremor with fairly good effect (Hildebrand and Delecluse 1987). It has also been used with some success to treat neuroleptic-induced EPS (Bersani et al. 1986).

The use of ritanserin in patients with schizophrenia has been explored in several small studies. By itself, it did not demonstrate antipsychotic activity, but it was thought to be helpful in the treatment of negative symptoms. In combination with haloperidol, there was some evidence that ritanserin reduced negative symptoms and EPS (Bersani et al. 1986; Duinkerke et al. 1993).

Other agents with 5-HT_2 antagonist properties, such as cyproheptadine, have been investigated as possible adjunct treatments. One open trial (Silver et al. 1989) demonstrated that cyproheptadine in combination with haloperidol was effective in reducing symptoms of schizophrenia. However, in a subsequent double-blind study, this effect was not shown (Silver et al. 1991). Cyproheptadine is not as specific a 5-HT_2 antagonist agent as ritanserin. Therefore, some of its other pharmacological properties (e.g., antihistamine) may have contributed to the clinical efficacy noted in the first trial. Several other 5-HT_2-specific agents have been examined for antipsychotic efficacy (mianserin and amperozide), but none has become accepted for general use (Axelsson et al. 1991; Mizuki et al. 1990).

Risperidone

The efficacy and lack of EPS of 5-HT_2 antagonists (such as ritanserin) in the treatment of schizophrenia led to the development of risperidone: 3-{2-[4-(6-fluoro-1,2-benzisoxazol-3-yl)-1-piperidinyl] ethyl}-6,7,8,9-tetrahydro-2-methyl-4*H*-pyridol[1,2-a]pyrimidin-4-one (see Figure 2–1). Risperidone combines both D_2 and potent 5-HT_2 antagonism (see Table 2–1).

Preclinical Pharmacological Studies

Risperidone induces catalepsy (the rodent equivalent of human EPS) at 20 times the corresponding dose of haloperidol (Janssen et al. 1988). Radioligand-receptor binding, neurotransmitter uptake assays, and ex vivo drug receptor dissociation rates demonstrate that the relative receptor affinity of risperidone for 5-HT_2 receptors is slightly higher than that of ritanserin (Leysen et al.

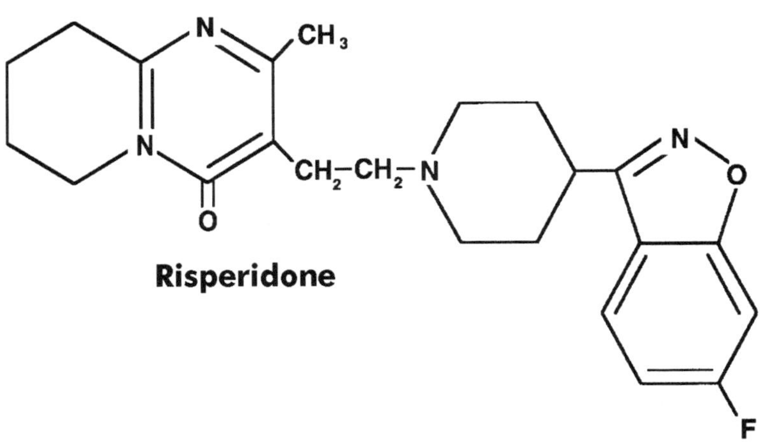

Figure 2–1. Chemical structure of risperidone. *Source.* Reprinted from Leysen JE, Gommeren W, Eens A, et al: "Biochemical Profile of Risperidone, a New Antipsychotic." *The Journal of Pharmacology and Experimental Therapeutics* 247:661–670, 1988. Used with permission.

Table 2–1. Receptor-binding profiles for risperidone, ritanserin, and haloperidol: results of two types of studies

		Risperidone	Ritanserin	Haloperidol
Receptor binding				
5-HT_2	a	9.29 ± 0.17	9.03 ± 0.20	7.09 ± 0.14
	b	0.16 ± 0.08	0.30 ± 0.13	25.1 ± 7.6
5-HT_{1a}	a	6.40 ± 0.08	5.54 ± 0.13	5.35 ± 0.23
	b	253 ± 47	1,370 ± 410	3,080 ± 1,680
5-HT_{1b}	a	< 5	< 5	
Dopamine-D_2	a	8.13 ± 0.18	7.42 ± 0.30	8.43 ± 0.16
	b	3.13 ± 1.30	30 ± 23	1.55 ± 0.47
Dopamine-D_1	a	6.07 ± 0.08	5.90 ± 0.11	6.45 ± 0.07
	b	534 ± 164	718 ± 187	255 ± 41
α_1 Adrenergic	a	8.66 ± 0.08	7.03 ± 0.13	7.45 ± 0.10
	b	0.81 ± 0.14	35.7 ± 9.5	10.9 ± 2.9
α_2 Adrenergic	a	7.70 ± 0.06	6.83 ± 0.12	< 6
	b	7.54 ± 1.00	56.4 ± 15.9	
β Adrenergic	a	< 5	< 5	< 5
Histamine-H_1	a	8.30 ± 0.01	7.48 ± 0.13	5.88 ± 0.04
	b	2.23 ± 0.11	11.8 ± 3.7	593 ± 48
Cholinergic-muscarinic	a	< 5	< 5	< 5
μ-Opiate	a	< 5	5.08 ± 0.04	5.45 ± 0.07
	b		1,740 ± 140	737 ± 120
Ca^{++} channel nitrendipine site	a	< 5	6.15 ± 0.05	5.80 ± 0.07
	b		496 ± 57	1,110 ± 180
Benzodiazepine	a	< 5	< 5	< 5
Substance P	a	< 5	< 5	< 5
Neurotensin	a	< 5	< 5	< 5
Release site	a	6.94 ± 0.10	6.10 ± 0.10	6.40 ± 0.10
	b	108 ± 22	750 ± 170	375 ± 90
Monoamine uptake				
Serotonin	a	6.23 ± 0.10	6.20 ± 0.14	6.08 ± 0.04
Norepinephrine	a	5.60 ± 0.07	6.32 ± 0.24	6.10 ± 0.14
Dopamine	a	5.32 ± 0.03	6.63 ± 0.04	5.80 ± 0.07
γ-Aminobutyric acid	a	< 5	5.58 ± 0.10	< 5

Note. a = $-\log [IC_{50}(M)]$ represents the potency of a drug to inhibit the uptake of neurotransmitters. Higher numbers indicate higher potencies. b = binding studies and the numbers are K_is (nM). The lower the K_i, the higher the affinity. Lower numbers indicate more potent binding to the receptor.

1988). Risperidone's relative receptor affinity for D_2 receptors is roughly one-half that of haloperidol. However, in vivo studies show that risperidone is 2.5 times more potent than haloperidol in antagonism of apomorphine-induced emesis in dogs. This is considered to be a peripheral effect mediated by D_2 receptors (Janssen et al. 1988). The discrepancies between in vitro and in vivo studies of the DA receptor potencies might have several explanations. There may be interspecies differences in brain penetration, or there may be other possible receptor affinities of risperidone that control emesis, such as 5-HT_3 antagonism (McBain et al. 1992).

Both ritanserin and risperidone dissociate slowly from 5-HT_2 receptors in vitro. In human platelets, they potently block serotonin-stimulated phosphoinositol formation and show no agonist potential. Of note, however, is that both drugs have some affinity for serotonin reuptake sites. Drug discrimination studies with rats demonstrate that risperidone is a potent and complete antagonist of lysergic acid diethylamide (LSD). Other drugs that demonstrate LSD antagonism include ritanserin, pirenperone, and setoperone (Ceulemans et al. 1985; Colpaert and Janssen 1983).

Pharmacokinetics and Metabolism

The pharmacokinetics and metabolism of risperidone and its active metabolite 9-hydroxyrisperidone (9-OH) have been studied in healthy volunteers and psychiatric patients (Heykants 1993). 9-OH has similar pharmacological activity to risperidone except that it is slightly less potent at the 5-HT_2 site. The pharmacokinetics of risperidone were studied after intravenous or oral administration in 12 dextromethorphan-phenotyped volunteers without psychosis. These volunteers were categorized as extensive (EM, n = 9), intermediate (IM, n = 1), or poor metabolizers (PM, n = 2) of debrisoquine. Europeans and North Americans comprise 5%–10% PMs. One percent of Asians are PMs. Risperidone's half-life was about 3 hours in the EMs and about 19 hours in the PMs. EMs' clearance rates were about seven times higher than that of PMs. Volumes of distribution did not differ between subjects. 9-OH plasma levels were higher in EMs, and, thus, they compensated for their more rapid risperidone elimination. Consequently, plasma concentrations of risperidone plus 9-OH were similar in all subjects, independent of their metabolic ratio. The elimination half-life of risperidone plus 9-OH averaged 20 hours.

Risperidone was rapidly absorbed after oral administration, and the plasma level peaked at 1 hour. Absolute oral bioavailability was almost 70% for risperidone and 100% for 9-OH. Plasma levels of 9-OH dropped with a half-life of 20 hours in EMs and PMs. Pharmacokinetic studies performed in patients with psychosis revealed that risperidone (1–8 mg bid) has a linear pharmacokinetic profile. In most patients, steady state was reached within 1 day for risperidone and within 5 days for risperidone plus 9-OH.

After an oral dose of radiolabeled risperidone (1 mg), about 70% was excreted in urine and 12%–18% in feces. Less than 1% of the dose was excreted as unchanged risperidone in feces and 5%–30% in urine. Hydroxylation to 9-OH was the main metabolic pathway. This accounted for 8%–32% of the administered dose excreted in urine. Oxidative *N*-dealkylation accounted for 10%–13% of the dose. Hydroxylation at the 7-position produced the least abundant metabolite (1%–5% of the dose).

Clinical Studies in Humans

In this chapter, we review more than a dozen clinical studies on the safety and efficacy of risperidone in psychotic patients. The designs, patient populations, and major findings of these studies are summarized in Table 2–2. The number of patients who have received risperidone exceeds the number of patients in the studies reviewed in this chapter. This is because, as of March 1995, risperidone is available to the public in 34 countries.

The studies reviewed in this chapter reflect the findings for 2,380 patients. The studies ranged from open label ($n = 355$) to double blind ($n = 2{,}025$). Several studies included psychotic individuals who did not necessarily have a diagnosis of schizophrenia (Gelders 1989; Gelders et al. 1990; Mesotten et al. 1989; Roose et al. 1988). All the studies were carried out with inpatients but varied regarding whether the patients were chronically ill (hospitalized many months) with schizophrenia (Claus et al. 1992; Chouinard et al. 1993; Marder and Meibach 1994) or were experiencing an acute exacerbation of their illness (Borison et al. 1992). The studies published to date vary not only in patient samples,

Table 2–2. Clinical research findings with risperidone

Study	Design	Subjects	Findings
Roose et al. 1988	Open label, flexible dose; risperidone 1.5–10.5 mg/day; 3–56 weeks	17 psychotic patients with mixed diagnoses	11 responders at mean dose (4.5 mg); only one patient responding had EPS
Castelao et al. 1989	Open label, flexible dose; risperidone 0.5–5 mg bid; 4 weeks; 1-week placebo washout	20 patients with schizophrenia	Improvement in negative symptoms, thought disturbance, and anxiety-depression-hostility at 2 weeks; 10 patients treated for EPS
Meco et al. 1989	Single blind, placebo controlled; risperidone 2–6 mg/day; 4 weeks; adjunctive to typical antipsychotic medication	10 patients with chronic schizophrenia with TD	Risperidone treatment improved BPRS and SANS; TD not significantly modified
Mesotten et al. 1989	Open label, flexible dose; risperidone 10–25 mg/day; 4 weeks	17 psychotic patients with mixed diagnoses	Inverted U-shaped curve relationship for dose with CGI and negative symptoms; EPS occurred at higher doses; loss of efficacy above 15 mg/day

Gelders et al. 1990	Open label, flexible dose; risperidone 1–10 mg/day; 4 weeks (31 patients received adjunctive benzodiazepines)	61 psychotic patients with mixed diagnoses	Early response of negative symptoms (within 7 days); significant improvement in BPRS compared to baseline; four patients required EPS medications
De Wilde and Dierick 1991	Open label, flexible dose; risperidone up to 20 mg/day; 52 weeks; 1-week placebo washout	36 patients with schizophrenia	27 patients had 50% or greater improvement in BPRS (both positive and negative symptoms); decrease in EPS
Ishigooka 1991	Open label, flexible dose; risperidone 1–15 mg/day; 8 weeks	83 patients in 29 centers	Improvement in BPRS and negative symptoms; side effects (10%) of patients: EPS, akathisia, fatigue, sleepiness, insomnia
Mertens 1991	Open label, flexible dose; risperidone 2–20 mg/day; 52 weeks	111 patients with schizophrenia	Average dose 8.2 mg/day; therapeutic effect within 2 weeks; positive and negative symptoms improved; 22 patients developed EPS; other side effects: concentration difficulties, sedation, memory disturbance, sleep reduction, 2.1 kg mean weight increase

(continued)

Table 2–2. Clinical research findings with risperidone *(continued)*

Study	Design	Subjects	Findings
Borison et al. 1992	Double blind, placebo controlled; risperidone 2–10 mg/day; haloperidol 4–20 mg/day; 6 weeks; randomized 18-day dosage titration	36 patients with acute schizophrenia	Risperidone more effective than placebo, trend toward more effective than haloperidol; rapid onset of action (within 2 weeks); EPS greater for haloperidol patients than risperidone or placebo; risperidone suppressed TD better than haloperidol
Claus et al. 1992	Double blind, randomized; risperidone average 12 mg/day; haloperidol average 10 mg/day; 2-week run-in and 1-week placebo washout	44 inpatients with chronic schizophrenia	Risperidone equal in efficacy to haloperidol but had less EPS
Müller-Spahn et al. 1992	Double blind; risperidone 1, 4, 8, 12, 16 mg/day; haloperidol 10 mg/day; 8 weeks	1,362 patients with schizophrenia	4–8 mg most effective dose with less EPS than 10 mg haloperidol

Chouinard et al. 1993	Double blind, fixed dose, placebo controlled; risperidone 2, 6, 10, 16 mg/day; haloperidol 20 mg/day; 6 weeks	135 inpatients with chronic schizophrenia	6 mg risperidone more effective and less EPS than 20 mg haloperidol; both risperidone and haloperidol more effective than placebo; risperidone at 6 mg had no more EPS than placebo; positive and negative symptoms improved
Marder and Meibach 1994	Double blind, fixed dose, placebo controlled; risperidone 2, 6, 10, 16 mg/day; haloperidol 20 mg/day; 6 weeks	388 inpatients with schizophrenia	6 mg risperidone more effective and less EPS than 20 mg haloperidol; both risperidone and haloperidol more effective than placebo; risperidone at 6 mg had no more EPS than placebo; positive and negative symptoms improved

Note. EPS = extrapyramidal side effects, TD = tardive dyskinesia, BPRS = Brief Psychiatric Rating Scale (Overall and Gorham 1962), SANS = Scale for the Assessment of Negative Symptoms (Andreasen 1982), CGI = clinical global improvement (Guy 1976).

but also in the use of rating scales, dosages of medication, and adjunctive medication. In particular, in one open-label study, one-half of the patients received benzodiazepines throughout the study (Gelders et al. 1990).

Efficacy

Optimal dosage. Open-label studies are potentially limited by raters' bias that affects the interpretation of the data for efficacy. However, one early open-label study predicted the clinical efficacy that was later demonstrated in rigorous placebo and active controlled studies (Mesotten et al. 1989). Inverted U-shaped curve relationships between clinical global improvement (CGI; Guy 1976) and negative symptoms were seen in relation to drug dose. There was a loss of efficacy at 15 mg/day in this open-label study. A similar pattern was seen in the United States and Canadian (North American Trial) double-blind studies (Chouinard et al. 1993; Marder and Meibach 1994) (see Figures 2–2, 2–3, and 2–4).

It appears from the double-blind studies that the most effective dose of risperidone for the "average" patient is in the range of 4–8 mg. In the North American multicenter study, clinical improvement was defined as a 20% reduction in total Positive and Negative Symptom Scale (PANSS; Kay et al. 1987) score at end point. This improvement was seen in 22% of the placebo patients; 35% of the patients receiving 2 mg of risperidone, 57% receiving 6 mg, 40% receiving 10 mg, and 51% receiving 16 mg; and in 30% of the patients receiving 20 mg of haloperidol in the United States sample (Figure 2–5). The Canadian data were very similar; response rates were 50%, 72.7%, 36.4%, 50%, and 47.6% for the risperidone doses of 2, 6, 10, and 16 mg and the haloperidol dose of 20 mg, respectively.

Two doses of risperidone, 6 and 16 mg daily, were significantly superior to placebo on all measures. End point scores on the PANSS positive subscale were significantly lower in patients receiving 6, 10, and 16 mg of risperidone than in the placebo-treated patients. Negative symptoms, however, were significantly lower, relative to placebo, in patients receiving 6 and 16 mg of risperidone. Taken together, these efficacy data suggest that risperidone begins to exert an antipsychotic effect at about 2 mg,

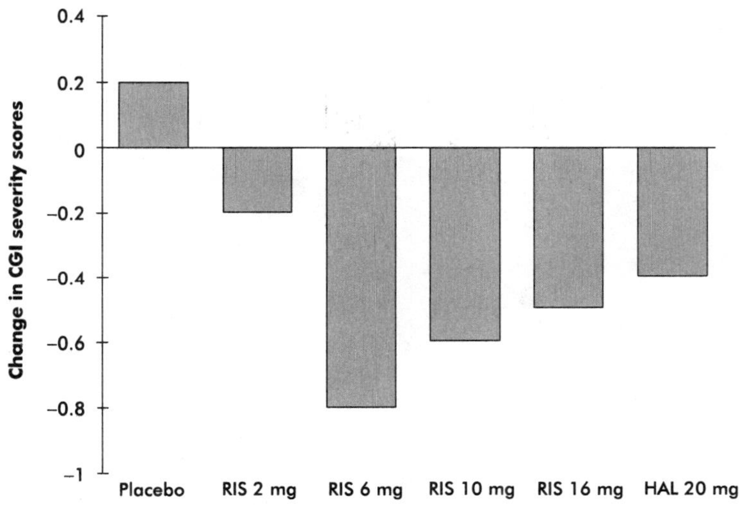

Figure 2–2. Average change in clinical global improvement (CGI) severity scores for patients in the North American double-blind trial of risperidone (RIS) versus placebo and haloperidol (HAL). *Source.* Reprinted from Marder SR, Meibach RC: "Risperidone in the Treatment of Schizophrenia." *American Journal of Psychiatry* 151:825–835, 1994. Copyright 1994, the American Psychiatric Association. Used with permission.

with a plateau in efficacy occurring at about 6 mg (see Figure 2–6). The dose response is then relatively flat until at least 16 mg—except for the curious "dip" in efficacy in the 10- to 12-mg range.

Onset of clinical improvement. Open-label and double-blind studies reflected a general trend of early onset of efficacy of risperidone. In the North American study, the median time to clinical improvement was 14 and 27 days for 6 and 16 mg of risperidone, respectively, versus 50 days in the placebo group and 29 days for patients receiving haloperidol. Time to clinical improvement was significantly shorter in the patients receiving 6 and 16 mg of risperidone than in those receiving placebo. The North American trial demonstrated a clear, significant ($P < .05$)

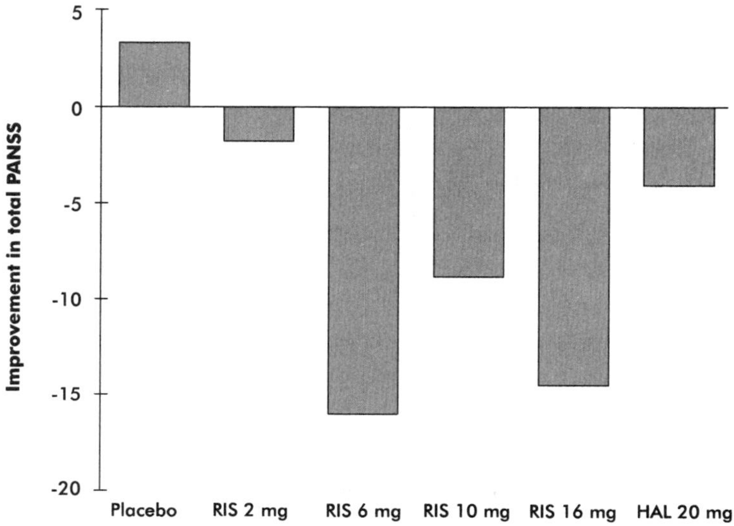

Figure 2–3. Average improvement in total score of the Positive and Negative Symptom Scale (PANSS) for patients in the North American double-blind trial of risperidone (RIS) versus placebo and haloperidol (HAL). *Source.* Reprinted from Marder SR, Meibach RC: "Risperidone in the Treatment of Schizophrenia." *American Journal of Psychiatry* 151:825–835, 1994. Copyright 1994, the American Psychiatric Association. Used with permission.

reduction in the total PANSS score within 7 days, which was maintained throughout the study for patients receiving the 6-mg dose of risperidone. This effect was seen within 14 days for the haloperidol-treated patients.

Clinical global improvement. When clinical improvement from baseline to end point was measured by the CGI, risperidone was found to be superior (at doses greater than 6 mg) to placebo. Improvement on the CGI (combining very much improved, much improved, and minimally improved) occurred in 29% of the placebo patients; in 44% of the patients receiving 2 mg of risperidone, 62% receiving 6 mg, 63% receiving 10 mg, and 65% receiving 16 mg; and in 48% of patients receiving haloperidol. The differ-

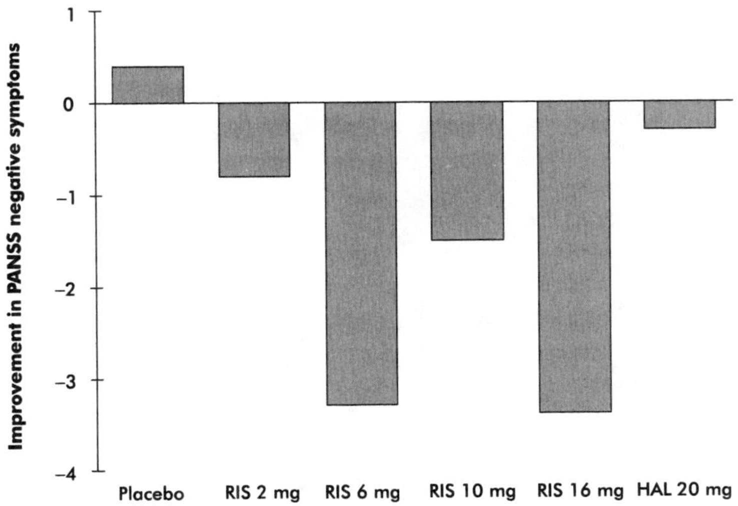

Figure 2–4. Average improvement in Positive and Negative Symptom Scale (PANSS) negative symptoms in the North American double-blind trial of risperidone (RIS) versus placebo and haloperidol (HAL). *Source.* Reprinted from Marder SR, Meibach RC: "Risperidone in the Treatment of Schizophrenia." *American Journal of Psychiatry* 151:825–835, 1994. Copyright 1994, the American Psychiatric Association. Used with permission.

ences between 6, 10, and 16 mg of risperidone versus placebo were significant ($P < .001$), as was the difference between haloperidol and placebo ($P < .01$) (Chouinard et al. 1993; Marder and Meibach 1994).

Positive and negative symptoms. In the North American trial, significant ($P < .01$) improvements from baseline to end point were obtained on all seven positive symptoms of the PANSS (delusions, conceptual disorganization, hallucinatory behavior, excitement, grandiosity, suspiciousness/persecution, and hostility) in patients receiving 6 mg of risperidone. In haloperidol-treated patients, significant improvements were noted in conceptual disorganization ($P < .01$), hallucinatory behavior ($P < .05$), and suspiciousness/persecution ($P < .01$). Changes in the total positive symptom score for all subjects are shown in

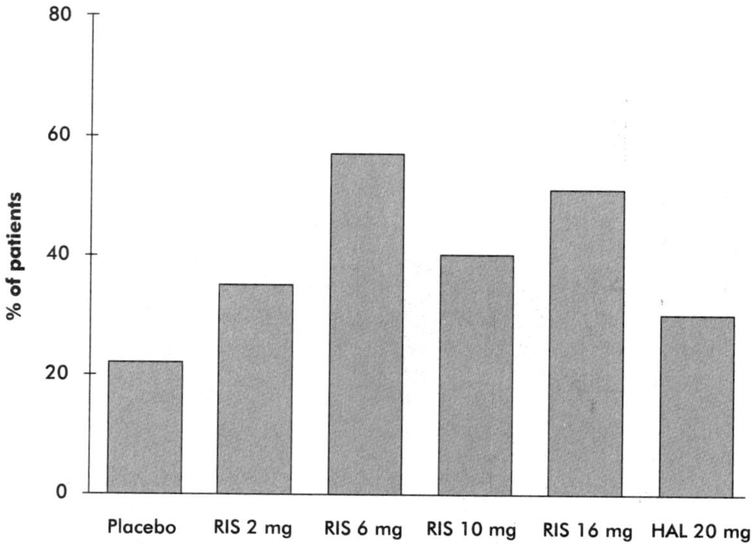

Figure 2–5. Percentage of patients achieving 20% or greater improvement on the Positive and Negative Symptom Scale. RIS = risperidone, HAL = haloperidol. *Source.* Reprinted from Marder SR, Meibach RC: "Risperidone in the Treatment of Schizophrenia." *American Journal of Psychiatry* 151:825–835, 1994. Copyright 1994, the American Psychiatric Association. Used with permission.

Figure 2–7. On the seven negative symptoms of the PANSS, patients receiving 6 mg of risperidone improved significantly from baseline on blunted affect ($P < .01$), emotional withdrawal ($P < .05$), poor rapport ($P < .05$), passive/apathetic social withdrawal ($P < .01$), difficulty in abstract thinking ($P < .01$), and stereotyped thinking ($P < .01$). Their scores on lack of spontaneity did not change significantly. No negative symptoms improved significantly from baseline in the patients receiving 20 mg of haloperidol.

Affective symptoms. Risperidone's efficacy for treating affective symptoms was examined in the 15-nation trial (Müller-Spahn et al. 1992; see "Fifteen-nation trial" subsection below). The sample was divided into a high anxiety/depression group and a

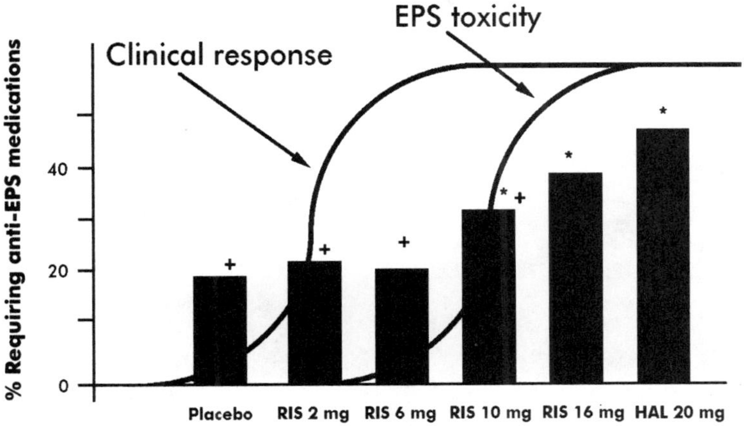

Figure 2–6. Percentage of patients receiving extrapyramidal side effect (EPS) medication in the North American double-blind trial of risperidone (RIS) versus placebo and haloperidol (HAL); histogram: idealized sigmoidal-shaped thresholds for both efficacy and neurotoxicity are drawn in. * = statistically more neurotoxicity than placebo, + = statistically less neurotoxicity than the 20-mg HAL group. *Source.* Reprinted from Marder SR, Meibach RC: "Risperidone in the Treatment of Schizophrenia." *American Journal of Psychiatry* 151:825–835, 1994. Copyright 1994, the American Psychiatric Association. Used with permission.

low anxiety/depression group based on subscales of the Brief Psychiatric Rating Scale (BPRS; Overall and Gorham 1962). In the high anxiety/depression patient group, risperidone 4–8 mg/day resulted in substantially better clinical improvement than haloperidol 10 mg/day. The North American trial demonstrated similar findings.

Comparison of Risperidone and Haloperidol

North American trial. The North American trial was designed to determine the most effective dose of risperidone relative to placebo. Because only a single dose of haloperidol (20 mg) was administered, these reports are not ideal for comparing the two active drugs. Nevertheless, interesting differences in the two

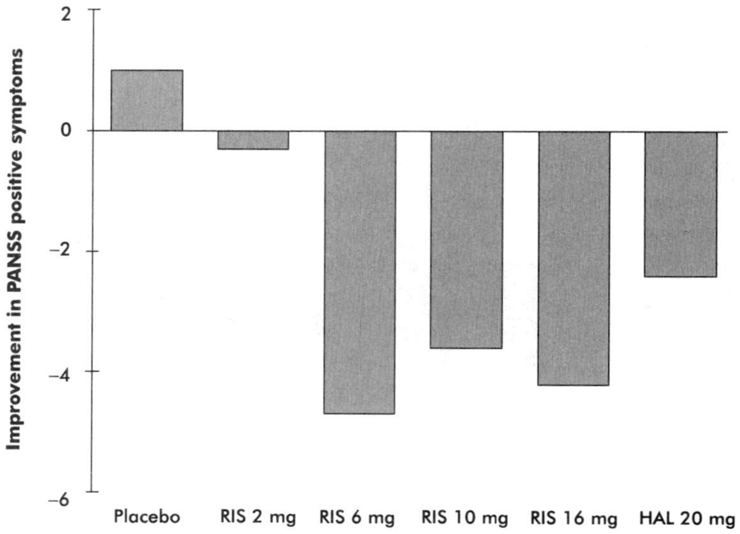

Figure 2–7. Average improvement in Positive and Negative Symptom Scale (PANSS) positive symptoms in the North American double-blind trial of risperidone (RIS) versus placebo and haloperidol (HAL). *Source.* Reprinted from Marder SR, Meibach RC: "Risperidone in the Treatment of Schizophrenia." *American Journal of Psychiatry* 151:825–835, 1994. Copyright 1994, the American Psychiatric Association. Used with permission.

drugs' efficacy were apparent. In the United States sample, significantly fewer patients receiving 20 mg of haloperidol were clinically improved, and they showed significantly smaller reductions in total PANSS scores than patients receiving 6 or 16 mg of risperidone (both $P < .05$). The Canadian study demonstrated similar findings. Risperidone at 6 mg resulted in a greater reduction in total PANSS score than haloperidol at 20 mg. Efficacy as measured by the CGI was significantly greater for patients receiving 6 mg of risperidone than haloperidol ($P < .05$) in both the United States and Canadian samples.

Fifteen-nation trial. Besides the North American study, a phase III comparison of haloperidol with risperidone was performed in a 15-nation study (13 European countries and 2 South American countries) that included 1,362 patients (Müller-Spahn et al. 1992; Peuskens et al. 1995). No placebo was used for comparison in this large sample. The doses of risperidone—1, 4, 8, 12, and 16 mg—were compared with 10 mg of haloperidol. The major efficacy findings from this trial were that there was a bell-shaped curve for the clinical response to risperidone (Figure 2–8). Optimal daily dose for therapeutic efficacy was 4–8 mg/day. This was greater than that of 1, 12, or 16 mg/day.

Extrapyramidal Side Effects

In the North American and Canadian trials, EPS induced by 6 mg of risperidone were virtually no different from those induced by placebo. As the dose increased to 16 mg, it was clear that the incidence of risperidone-induced EPS was greater than that of placebo. This was also true for haloperidol 20 mg (Chouinard et al.

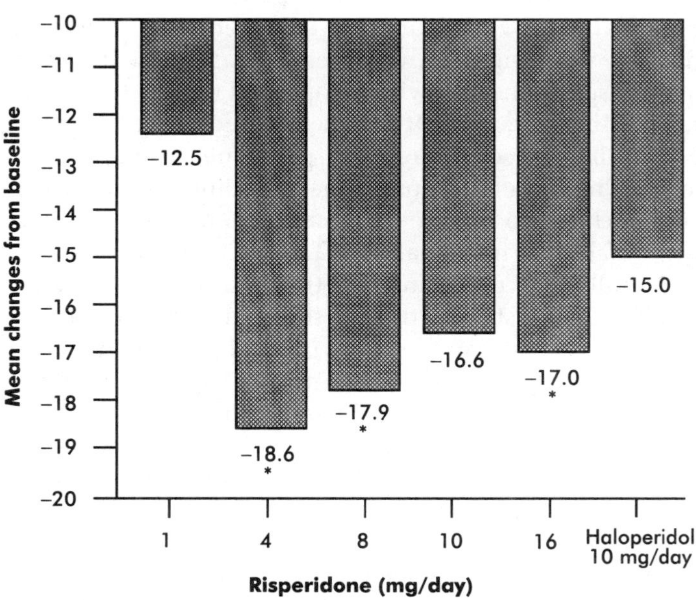

Figure 2–8. Fifteen-nation trial results: mean changes from baseline to end point in total Positive and Negative Symptom Scale scores. * = significantly better than 1 mg of risperidone.

1993; Marder and Meibach 1994). In the United States double-blind study, antiparkinsonian medication was given to 18% of the patients receiving placebo; to 22% of the patients receiving 2 mg of risperidone, 20% receiving 6 mg, 31% receiving 10 mg, and 39% receiving 16 mg; and to 47% receiving 20 mg of haloperidol (Figure 2–6). The Canadian study by Chouinard and colleagues showed similar percentages of patients requiring antiparkinsonian medication (25%, 31.8%, 45.5%, and 50% for risperidone 2, 6, 10, and 16 mg, respectively). Significant differences were noted between placebo and 16 mg of risperidone and 20 mg of haloperidol in both studies. Significantly fewer risperidone-treated patients received antiparkinsonian drugs than did haloperidol-treated patients except for those patients treated with 16 mg of risperidone.

The use of antiparkinsonian medication was an objective measure of EPS in these studies. The clinical assessments of EPS were made with the Extrapyramidal Symptom Rating Scale (ESRS; Chouinard et al. 1980). No significant differences in ESRS score changes were found between patients receiving placebo and patients receiving 2 or 6 mg of risperidone. Parkinsonian symptoms were significantly greater during treatment with 16 mg of risperidone and with haloperidol than with placebo. In summary, the suggestion of enhanced clinical efficacy and negligible EPS liability of the 6-mg risperidone dose are the most powerful findings of the North American clinical trial. It is tempting to conclude from these data that the 6-mg dose is therefore the "optimal" dose for all patients. This is clearly overly simplistic and clinically inaccurate. Instead, the data should be viewed as apparently demonstrating that the threshold for antipsychotic effect begins at (or perhaps before) 2 mg and that the threshold for neurotoxicity begins at about 10 mg (see Figure 2–6). Between these doses is a potential clinical window in which antipsychotic effect might be achieved with little or no EPS. Because these data were derived from a relatively homogeneous clinical group, it is likely that these general window parameters will be shifted, broadened, or narrowed for another patient group.

The 15-nation trial also demonstrated the low EPS liability of risperidone. Scores for dystonia and akathisia were less for all doses of risperidone than for haloperidol 10 mg/day ($P < .05$) (Lopez Ibor Alino 1992; Möller 1992; Müller-Spahn et al. 1992). EPS ratings for the 4-mg dose of risperidone were not significantly different from the 1-mg risperidone dose putative placebo control in this study. However, 8 mg of risperidone produced significantly more side effects than 1 mg of risperidone ($P < .05$) (Owens 1993). Scores on ratings of EPS were less for risperidone 4–8 mg/day than for haloperidol 10 mg/day ($P < .05$).

Other Safety Findings

The open-label and double-blind studies published to date reflect that risperidone is a very well-tolerated medication. No significant hematological side effects were reported in any of the studies. The most frequent side effects mentioned in the studies were agitation, anxiety, insomnia, EPS, headache, nausea, and drowsiness. Adverse events with a difference in incidence of more than 5% between placebo and 16 mg of risperidone included somnolence (reported by 0% of placebo patients versus 9.4% of patients receiving 16 mg of risperidone), EPS (10.6% versus 25%, respectively), dizziness (0% versus 10.9%, respectively), constipation (0% versus 6.3%, respectively), and tachycardia (0% versus 6.3%, respectively) (Marder and Meibach 1994).

In the North American trial (United States sample) the following side effects appeared to be correlated to the dose of risperidone: fatigue ($P < .05$), sedation ($P < .05$), accommodation disturbances ($P < .05$), orthostatic dizziness ($P < .05$), palpitations or tachycardia ($P < .01$), weight gain ($P < .05$), diminished sexual desire ($P < .05$), and erectile dysfunction ($P < .01$). No clinically significant abnormal laboratory test results were recorded in any of the risperidone-treated patients. The Canadian sample had similar results—agitation, anxiety, insomnia, headache, and nausea were the most frequently reported side effects. Syncope occurred in one patient on 10 mg of risperidone. Three patients experienced orthostatic tachycardia (6, 10, 16 mg of risperidone), one experienced hypotension (risperidone 16 mg), and one experienced postural hypotension (risperidone 6 mg) (Chouinard et al. 1993). Because of its potential to cause orthostatic hypotension, risperidone should be slowly titrated, in two divided doses. These events were all transient in nature and required no long-term treatment. A significant safety finding from the 15-nation trial was that serum prolactin increased in risperidone-treated patients. This is a well-known effect of D_2 antagonists. No significant changes were seen in blood pressure, heart rate, or electrocardiogram (Müller-Spahn et al. 1992).

Long-Term Studies

There has not been a great deal of long-term experience with risperidone. Currently, one long-term study has been reported involving 264 patients. They have received risperidone for a mean of 7.4 months (maximum 15.4 months) at a mean dose of 7.6 mg/day. An improvement has been noted in all five clusters of the BPRS scale (anergia, thought disorder, anxiety/depression, activity, and hostility). The total BPRS score decreased by at least 20% in 70% of these patients. In more than half of this sample, the investigator considered that the progress was much better or better than that achieved on the patients' previous medications (Mertens 1991, 1992). Another long-term study that lasted almost 13 months has demonstrated similar results (De Wilde and Dierick 1991).

Future Research

The studies of risperidone to date are promising. However, many questions still need to be answered regarding the clinical efficacy and safety of risperidone. For example, the long-term experience with the drug is limited at this point. Its effect on a patient's social adjustment, course of illness, and compliance is virtually unknown. More long-term treatment studies that focus on these outcome variables must be performed to answer these questions. In addition, we do not know how effective risperidone will be in certain clinical populations (e.g., treatment-resistant patients). The effectiveness of risperidone in patients with primarily negative symptoms also needs to be addressed. This leads to the question of whether risperidone will be more clinically effective and better tolerated than clozapine, a medication that has proven efficacy in treatment-resistant patients (Kane et al. 1988). We also do not know how effective risperidone may be in geriatric and bipolar-psychotic patients. Likewise, its long-term risk of causing tardive dyskinesia and its utility in first-break schizophrenia patients are unknown.

In summary, risperidone, thus far, appears to be a pharmacologically unique, safe, and effective medication. However, our clinical experience with this molecule is limited. We must investigate it further to broaden our knowledge and to improve the quality of life of patients with psychotic illnesses.

References

Andreasen NC: Negative symptoms in schizophrenia: definition and reliability. Arch Gen Psychiatry 39:784–788, 1982

Axelsson R, Nilsson A, Christensson E, et al: Effects of amperozide in schizophrenia: an open study of a potent 5-HT2 receptor agonist. Psychopharmacology 104:287–292, 1991

Benson KL, Kym FF, Zarcone VP Jr: Evidence for the role of serotonin in the regulation of slow wave sleep in schizophrenia. Sleep 14:133–139, 1991

Bersani G, Grispini A, Marini S, et al: Neuroleptic-induced extrapyramidal side effects: clinical perspectives with ritanserin (R55667), a new selective 5-HT2 receptor blocking agent. Current Therapeutic Research 40:492–499, 1986

Borison RL, Pathiraja AP, Diamond B, et al: Risperidone: clinical safety and efficacy in schizophrenia. Psychopharmacol Bull 28:213–218, 1992

Castelao JF, Ferreira L, Gelders YG, et al: The efficacy of the D_2 and 5-HT_2 antagonist risperidone (R64 766) in the treatment of chronic psychosis: an open dose-finding study. Schizophr Res 2:411–415, 1989

Ceulemans DLS, Gelders YG, Hoppenbrouwers M-LJA, et al: Effect of serotonin antagonism in schizophrenia: a pilot study with setoperone. Psychopharmacology 85:329–332, 1985

Chouinard G, Ross-Chouinard A, Annable L, et al: Extrapyramidal Symptom Rating Scale (abstract). Can J Neurol Sci 7:233, 1980

Chouinard G, Jones B, Remington G, et al: A Canadian multicenter placebo-controlled study of fixed doses of risperidone and haloperidol in the treatment of chronic schizophrenic patients. J Clin Psychopharmacol 13:25–40, 1993

Claus A, Bollen J, De Cuyper H, et al: Risperidone versus haloperidol in the treatment of chronic schizophrenic inpatients: a multicentre double-blind comparative study. Acta Psychiatr Scand 85:295–305, 1992

Colpaert FC, Janssen PAJ: A characterization of LSD-antagonist effect pirenperone in the rat. Neuropharmacology 22:1001–1005, 1983

Declerck AC, Wauquier A, Van Der Ham-Veltman PHM, et al: Increase in slow-wave sleep in humans with the serotonin-S2 antagonist ritanserin: the first exploratory polygraphic sleep study. Current Therapeutic Research 41:427–432, 1987

De Wilde J, Dierick M: Long-term treatment of schizophrenic patients with risperidone (abstract). Biol Psychiatry 1:675S, 1991

Duinkerke SJ, Botter PA, Jansen AI, et al: Ritanserin, a selective 5-HT2/1c antagonist, and negative symptoms in schizophrenia: a placebo-controlled double-blind trial. Br J Psychiatry 163:451–455, 1993

Farde L, Norstrom A-L, Wiesel F-A, et al: Positron emission tomographic analysis of central D1 and D2 dopamine receptor occupancy in patients treated with classical neuroleptics and clozapine: relation to extrapyramidal side effects. Arch Gen Psychiatry 49:538–544, 1992

Gelders YG: Thymosthenic agents, a novel approach in the treatment of schizophrenia. Br J Psychiatry 144 (suppl 5):33–36, 1989

Gelders YG, Heylen SLE, Vanden Bussche G, et al: Pilot clinical investigation of risperidone in the treatment of psychotic patients. Pharmacopsychiatry 23:206–211, 1990

Guy W (ed): ECDEU Assessment Manual for Psychopharmacology, Revised (DHEW Publ No ADM 76-338). Rockville, MD, U.S. Department of Health, Education and Welfare, 1976

Heykants JJP: The pharmacokinetics of risperidone in man. Paper presented at the 9th World Congress of Psychiatry, Rio de Janeiro, Brazil, June 6–12, 1993

Hildebrand J, Delecluse F: Effect of ritanserin, a selective serotonin-S2 antagonist, on parkinsonian rest tremor. Current Therapeutic Research 41:298–300, 1987

Idzikowski C, Mills FJ, Glennard R: 5-hydroxytryptamine-2 antagonist increases human slow wave sleep. Brain Res 378:164–168, 1986

Ishigooka J: Clinical experience with risperidone in Japan—a multicentre early phase II trial, in Risperidone: Major Progress in Antipsychotic Treatment. Edited by Kane JM. Oxford, England, Oxford Clinical Communications, 1991, pp 40–43

Janssen PAJ: The relevance of pharmacological studies to sleep research in psychiatry. Pharmacopsychiatry 21:33–37, 1988

Janssen PA, Niemegeers CJ, Awouters F, et al: Pharmacology of risperidone (R 64 766), a new antipsychotic with serotonin-S2 and dopamine-D2 antagonistic properties. J Pharmacol Exp Ther 244:685–693, 1988

Jouvet M: Biogenic amines and the stages of sleep. Science 163:391–399, 1969

Kane J, Honigfeld G, Singer J, et al: Clozapine for the treatment-resistant schizophrenic: a double-blind comparison with chlorpromazine. Arch Gen Psychiatry 45:789–796, 1988

Kay SR, Fiszbein A, Opler LA: The Positive and Negative Symptom Scale (PANSS) for schizophrenia. Schizophr Bull 13:261–276, 1987

Leysen JE, Gommeren W, Eens A, et al: Biochemical profile of risperidone, a new antipsychotic. J Pharmacol Exp Ther 247:661–670, 1988

Lopez Ibor Alino JJ: Risperidone: safety and side-effect profile. Paper presented at the First International Risperidone Investigators' Meeting, Paris, France, March 9–10, 1992

Marder SR, Meibach RC: Risperidone in the treatment of schizophrenia. Am J Psychiatry 151:825–835, 1994

McBain SL, Dineen M, Weller M, et al: Odansetron, a double blind placebo controlled study in acute schizophrenia. Paper presented at the VIth Biennial European Workshop on Schizophrenia, Badgastein, Austria, January 26–31, 1992

Meco G, Bedini L, Bonifati V, et al: Risperidone in the treatment of chronic schizophrenia with tardive dyskinesia: a single-blind crossover study versus placebo. Current Therapeutic Research 46:876–883, 1989

Meltzer HY: Duration of a clozapine trial in neuroleptic-resistant schizophrenia (letter). Arch Gen Psychiatry 46:672, 1989

Meltzer HY, Matsubara S, Lee J-C: Classification of typical and atypical antipsychotic drugs on the basis of dopamine D-1, and D-2 and serotonin2 pKi values. J Pharmacol Exp Ther 251:238–246, 1989

Mertens C: Long-term treatment of chronic schizophrenic patients with risperidone, in Risperidone: Major Progress in Antipsychotic Treatment. Edited by Kane JM. Oxford, England, Oxford Clinical Communications, 1991, pp 44–48

Mertens C: Long-term experience with risperidone. Paper presented at the First International Risperidone Investigators' Meeting, Paris, France, March 9–10, 1992

Mesotten F, Suy E, Pietquin M, et al: Therapeutic effect and safety of increasing doses of risperidone (R 64766) in psychotic patients. Psychopharmacology 99:445–449, 1989

Mizuki Y, Kajimura N, Imai T, et al: Effects of mianserin on negative symptoms in schizophrenia. Int Clin Psychopharmacol 5:83–95, 1990

Möller HJ: Incidence of EPS under risperidone therapy. Paper presented at the First International Risperidone Investigators' Meeting, Paris, France, March 9–10, 1992

Müller-Spahn F, The International Risperidone Research Group: Risperidone in the treatment of chronic schizophrenic patients: an international double-blind parallel-group study versus haloperidol. Clin Neuropharmacol 15 (suppl 1):90A–91A, 1992

Overall JE, Gorham DR: The Brief Psychiatric Rating Sale. Psychol Rep 10:799–812, 1962

Owens DGC: Extrapyramidal side effects and general tolerability of risperidone. Paper presented at the 9th World Congress of Psychiatry, Rio de Janeiro, Brazil, June 6–12, 1993

Peuskens J, on behalf of the Risperidone Study Group: Risperidone in the treatment of patients with chronic schizophrenia: a multi-national, multi-centre, double-blind, parallel-group study versus haloperidol. Br J Psychiatry 166:712–726, 1995

Reyntjens A, Gelders YG, Hoppenbrouwers M-LJA, et al: Thymosthenic effects of ritanserin (R 55667), a centrally acting serotonin-S2 receptor blocker. Drug Development Research 8:205–211, 1986

Roose K, Gelders Y, Heylen S: Risperidone (R64 766) in psychotic patients: a first clinical therapeutic exploration. Acta Psychiatr Belg 88:233–241, 1988

Seeman P, Lee T, Chau Wong M, et al: Antipsychotic drug doses and neuroleptic/dopamine receptors. Nature 261:717–719, 1976

Silver H, Blacker M, Weller MPI, et al: Treatment of chronic schizophrenia with cyproheptadine. Biol Psychiatry 25:502–504, 1989

Silver H, Blacker M, Weller MPI, et al: Treatment of chronic schizophrenia with cyproheptadine: a double-blind placebo-controlled study. Biol Psychiatry 30:523–525, 1991

Ugedo L, Grenhoff J, Svensson TH: Ritanserin, a 5HT2 receptor antagonist activates midbrain dopamine neurons by blocking serotonergic inhibition. Psychopharmacology 98:45–50, 1989

Van Putten T: Why do schizophrenic patients refuse to take their drugs? Arch Gen Psychiatry 31:67–72, 1974

CHAPTER 3

Future Antipsychotic Agents: Clinical Implications

Anil K. Malhotra, M.D.
Debra A. Pinsky, M.D.
Alan Breier, M.D.

The introduction of clozapine in the United States marked the first major breakthrough in the pharmacotherapy of schizophrenia since the introduction of chlorpromazine 40 years earlier. Clozapine is the first antipsychotic agent that is not associated with extrapyramidal side effects (EPS) or tardive dyskinesia, and double-blind, placebo-controlled drug trials have shown it to be more effective than typical neuroleptics in chronically symptomatic schizophrenic patients (Kane et al. 1988; Pickar et al. 1992).

This extraordinary clinical profile of superior efficacy and lack of EPS has provided a new model for antipsychotic treatment. This "New Pharmacotherapy of Schizophrenia" has been inspired by the pressing need for medications that offer more clinical benefits than the traditional neuroleptics used for the past 40 years. Many novel agents are being developed that we hope will meet this demand. We must determine what characteristics these new drugs should contain and how to evaluate these medications as they become available.

The New Pharmacotherapy of Schizophrenia

Improved Antipsychotic Efficacy

Several issues must be addressed by pharmaceutical companies hoping to provide new agents with significant improvements over previous treatments (Table 3–1). First, novel agents that provide improved antipsychotic efficacy over typical neuroleptics will be of great benefit. Despite treatment, schizophrenia remains a disabling illness that often renders the patient unemployable, unable to maintain social relationships, and prone to depressive episodes and suicide (Roy 1982). So-called treatment-responsive patients often still hear voices or have other disorders of perception, whereas a significant subset of patients do not even achieve this level of symptom relief. If the new pharmacotherapy can improve treatment response, these drugs will offer real hope for millions of patients around the globe.

Lack of Extrapyramidal Side Effects and Tardive Dyskinesia

The new pharmacotherapy also hopes to extend the experience of clozapine and develop other antipsychotic agents that are not associated with EPS and tardive dyskinesia. The clinical implications of this are enormous. Patients will be more likely to comply with treatment regimens, may appear to have fewer negative symptoms, and will be free of concerns about developing a potentially irreversible movement disorder. This will allow for more effective treatment and should markedly improve the quality of life of many patients.

Table 3–1. Goals of future new pharmacotherapeutic agents for schizophrenia

Improved antipsychotic efficacy
Decreased extrapyramidal side effects
Decreased propensity to induce tardive dyskinesia
Efficacy for negative symptoms
Enhanced functioning and quality of life

To achieve this important goal, psychopharmacological researchers can utilize animal models of psychosis and EPS to screen for potentially useful compounds. In one model, a drug's ability to inhibit amphetamine-induced stereotypies may indicate antipsychotic efficacy, whereas induction of catalepsy represents a drug's propensity for EPS. Validation of this model is provided by clozapine's decreased ability to produce catalepsy in laboratory animals compared with typical neuroleptics (Meltzer 1990). Another useful preclinical model is derived from clozapine's selectivity for specific regions in rat brain corresponding to human brain areas thought to be involved in antipsychotic efficacy and neurological side effects. Chronic administration of clozapine to the rat produces a decrease in dopamine neuron firing in ventral tegmental area (A10), a putative limbic site involved in psychotic phenomena, and produces limited effects on nigrostriatal (A9) regions responsible for neurological effects. Typical neuroleptics, on the other hand, suppress firing in both of these regions (Chiodo and Bunney 1983). These findings may help explain why clozapine maintains the therapeutic efficacy of typical neuroleptics without the associated EPS or tardive dyskinesia and represents another useful preclinical screen for *atypical* antipsychotics.

Treatment of Negative Symptoms

A third hallmark of the new pharmacotherapy of schizophrenia is the emphasis on better treatments for the negative symptoms (i.e., alogia, apathy, anhedonia, blunted affect). The negative symptoms often represent the real stumbling blocks for patients trying to lead more fruitful and satisfying lives. Several studies have suggested that long-term outcome for patients with schizophrenia is associated with negative symptomatology (Breier et al. 1991; Fenton and McGlashan 1994). Although early reports suggested that clozapine has superior efficacy for negative symptoms, more recent studies suggest that this finding may actually be related to clozapine's lack of EPS (W. T. Carpenter et al. 1995). Novel agents that provide true relief from this subset of schizophrenic symptomatology will offer substantial benefits to the large number of patients who primarily endure these important, although often underappreciated, set of symptoms.

Improvements in Overall Functioning and Quality of Life

Finally, the new pharmacotherapy may use additional parameters to establish a drug's therapeutic efficacy than those previously used. To complement standardized rating scales that quantify precise levels of particular symptoms, it is often informative to make assessments of a more global nature. With clozapine, it seems clear that treated patients' quality of life, as measured by social and work functioning, continues to improve long after the standard 6–8 weeks of a drug trial. In fact, some studies have shown that these global improvements continue up to a year after initiation of treatment (Breier et al. 1993). Whether these marked improvements are due to clozapine's resultant reduction in psychotic symptoms, its favorable side-effect profile, or its apparent efficacy for secondary negative symptoms is not clear. Nevertheless, the new antipsychotic agents hope to provide superior or equivalent levels of improvement in these areas, and quality of life measurements may ultimately prove to be more useful and, perhaps, more relevant to the patients undergoing treatment.

New Antipsychotic Medications

Many novel antipsychotic agents are currently being developed for general use in the United States (Table 3–2). The following potential antipsychotic agents represent a small number of those

Table 3–2. Promising new antipsychotic agents

			Action			
Agent	Phase	FDA-approved	Dopamine D_2	Serotonin $5\text{-}HT_2$	Noradrenergic α_2	Muscarinic
Clozapine	IV	1989	+	++	+	+++
Risperidone	IV	1993	+++	+++	++	+
Sertindole	III		+++	+++	±	+
Olanzapine	III		++	++	++	++
Seroquel	III		+	+	+++	+

Note. ± = no to low affinity; + = low affinity; ++ = moderate affinity; +++ = high affinity.

currently being investigated. This abbreviated list highlights the pharmacotherapeutic strategies used in the development of ideal antipsychotic agents.

Risperidone

Most recently, risperidone was approved by the Food and Drug Administration (FDA) for the treatment of schizophrenia. Risperidone is the first novel antipsychotic agent since clozapine to be made available in the United States and only the second since 1975. Risperidone's clinical profile is examined in Chapter 2 in this volume.

Risperidone's mechanism of action is unknown. Like clozapine, it antagonizes 5-HT_2 receptors as well as other neurochemical systems (Janssen et al. 1988). However, it differs from clozapine in having much greater binding affinity at both the 5-HT_2 and D_2 receptors. Its greater D_2 affinity may explain its dose-dependent effects of producing EPS. Preclinically, risperidone has been shown to inhibit apomorphine-induced stereotypies and to produce catalepsy at only higher doses (Chouinard et al. 1993; Janssen et al. 1988).

The preliminary data from preclinical and clinical studies of risperidone are hopeful. Risperidone is an effective antipsychotic, may be more efficacious in the treatment of negative symptoms than traditional neuroleptics, and produces a lesser degree of EPS than the typical neuroleptics when used in the lower dosage ranges (Borison et al. 1992; Chouinard et al. 1993). Its effects on quality of life over the long term are unknown; however, it is encouraging that this drug does not require the intensive monitoring that clozapine does. Three clinical questions remain unanswered: 1) Is risperidone a superior treatment for treatment-resistant schizophrenia? 2) Does risperidone have superior efficacy compared with traditional neuroleptics? and 3) Does increasing the dose above 6 mg/day in nonresponders lead to improved efficacy? Studies are currently under way to address these issues.

Sertindole

Sertindole is another compound that has aroused interest as a potential atypical antipsychotic. Early phase III studies in the

United States have demonstrated antipsychotic efficacy superior to that of placebo and comparable to that of haloperidol without producing EPS in patients with schizophrenia who have histories of neuroleptic response. Preclinical studies demonstrating preferential blockade of mesolimbic neurons suggest a lack of associated EPS, although mild motor effects, including tremor, have been reported (Skarsfeldt and Perregaard 1990). Initial studies have shown that sertindole produces cardiovascular side effects, including orthostatic hypotension, tachycardia, and syncope, although tolerance to these side effects may develop.

Sertindole's pharmacological profile is of note because it has high potencies at both D_2 and 5-HT_2 receptors and is therefore similar to risperidone. This, in addition to reports of motor side effects, raises the question as to whether sertindole is truly atypical because high levels of D_2 blockade have been correlated with EPS. Sertindole, therefore, will require further evaluation before gaining approval as an atypical antipsychotic agent.

Olanzapine

Olanzapine is a thienobenzodiazepine with antipsychotic potential. Preliminary open-label and blinded studies have demonstrated significant reductions in psychotic symptoms without associated EPS. Adverse side effects appear to be minimal and include sedation, dizziness, constipation, and nausea (Tollefson et al. 1994). Because olanzapine has only been tested in a limited number of patients, further studies are required to determine the incidence and significance of these side effects.

Olanzapine has a favorable preclinical profile with potent 5-HT_2-antagonist activity and a lesser affinity for dopaminergic receptors. Some studies have reported the affinity of olanzapine to 5-HT_2 receptors to be more than twice as high as the affinity for D_2 receptors (Fuller and Snoddy 1992). Preclinical studies further demonstrate reductions in apomorphine-induced climbing and avoidance behaviors in rats at doses much lower than those used to induce catalepsy (Moore et al. 1992).

Olanzapine, then, is another promising atypical agent. If future studies confirm this clinical profile, olanzapine may soon be available for general use in the United States.

ICI 204,636 (Seroquel)

The investigational agent ICI 204,636 (Seroquel) represents another promising antipsychotic medication. Initial clinical research demonstrated a significant decrease in Brief Psychiatric Rating Scale (BPRS; Overall and Gorham 1962) scores in mild to moderately ill patients with chronic schizophrenia. Most important, ICI 204,636 has not been reported to produce EPS or acute dystonic reactions. Side effects have included transient cardiovascular effects such as sinus tachycardia, sedation, and insomnia (Fabre et al. 1990).

ICI 204,636 is a dibenzothiazepine with high 5-HT_2 affinity combined with some affinity for D_2 receptors. Consistent with its reported decreased propensity to induce EPS, ICI 204,636 has been shown in animal studies preferentially to affect dopaminergic pathways associated with psychosis more than those associated with EPS (Malick et al. 1990).

It is clear that further investigation of ICI 204,636 is warranted. Its clinical efficacy and lack of EPS are encouraging. It remains to be seen whether this compound will offer improved antipsychotic efficacy over traditional neuroleptics; provide improved treatment of negative symptoms; or, in the long term, have substantial effects on the quality of life of patients. If so, this drug will be a welcome addition to the new pharmacotherapy of schizophrenia.

Amperozide

Amperozide is another new atypical antipsychotic agent. It has been tested in phase II clinical trials in a limited number of patients with schizophrenia (Axelsson et al. 1991; Mertens et al. 1989). In these studies, more than 60% of patients showed significant improvement from baseline scores of psychotic symptoms at doses ranging from 5 to 20 mg/day. Nine patients had no clinical response in the study by Mertens et al. (1989), and one patient was noted to have a worsening of psychotic symptoms in the study by Axelsson et al. (1991). Amperozide, with its potent 5-HT_2-receptor antagonist properties and almost no D_2-receptor antagonism, raises the question of whether a drug with these biochemical properties will be significantly effective for the treatment of schizophrenia.

Doses used in early studies were less than 20 mg/day; higher doses led to more pronounced side effects, but these were minimal and reported inconsistently. The side effects of most concern were electrocardiogram (ECG) changes, including prolonged Q-Tc interval and T-wave flattening (Axelsson et al. 1991). Other common side effects of less concern included nausea, drowsiness, anxiety, and dizziness. Rare reports of diaphoresis, blurred vision, congestion, mouth stiffness, dry mouth, and decreased sleep have also been noted (Axelsson et al. 1991; Mertens et al. 1989).

EPS secondary to treatment with amperozide are minimal. Of these, tremor was observed most frequently. Rigidity (found to be unresponsive to standard anticholinergics in one severe case reported) and sialorrhea were also seen (Axelsson et al. 1991). Further studies are needed to determine the significance of these findings.

A great deal of research has been done to understand amperozide's precise mechanism of action. Amperozide has not been shown to be a potent D_2 antagonist, but it is a potent 5-HT_2-receptor antagonist with lesser affinities to α_1- and α_2-adrenergic receptors (Christensson and Bjork 1990; Meltzer et al. 1992; Svartengren and Simonsson 1990). Some investigators have suggested that amperozide acts presynaptically to modulate dopamine release, reuptake, and turnover (Christensson and Gustafsson 1985; Meltzer et al. 1992). This mechanism, rather than striatal and limbic blockade of D_2 receptors, may account for amperozide's clinical profile and decreased association with EPS.

Preliminary data, then, suggest that amperozide may be an effective antipsychotic agent; however, further investigation is necessary to clarify amperozide's clinical profile and mechanism of action. If amperozide does prove successful, traditional hypotheses about dopaminergic blockade and antipsychotic efficacy will require fundamental reevaluation.

Remoxipride

A cautionary note, however, has resulted from recent experience with remoxipride. Remoxipride is a substituted benzamide studied extensively for its antipsychotic properties. In double-blind comparisons with haloperidol, remoxipride has been shown to be effective in the treatment of the positive and negative symptoms of schizophrenia (Chouinard 1987; Lewander et al. 1990). In a combined analysis of nine double-blind studies comparing remoxipride with haloperidol, Lewander et al. (1990) reported significant improvements in 57% of 500 patients treated with remoxipride (150–600 mg/day) and in 57% of 358 patients treated with haloperidol (5–45 mg/day). In addition, this study reported that 40%–45% of the remoxipride-treated patients experienced a greater than 50% reduction in total BPRS score. The results of other studies were not as promising. For example, in a study by Chouinard (1990), remoxipride did not compare favorably to chlorpromazine.

Remoxipride was not associated with any significant EPS or tardive dyskinesia (Chouinard 1987; Lewander et al. 1990). In comparison to haloperidol, remoxipride has been associated with a lower incidence of sedation, blurred vision, and dry mouth (Lewander et al. 1990). Cardiovascular side effects were seen infrequently and included minor ECG changes and some reports of postural hypotension, dizziness, and either increased or decreased heart rate (Chouinard 1987).

Remoxipride's mechanism of action and limited side-effect profile may be due to its neuropharmacological and neuroanatomical profile. Remoxipride is a weak but selective central D_2 antagonist with low affinities for cholinergic, serotonergic, histamine, muscarinic, or α_1-adrenergic receptors (Wadworth and Heel 1990). The dose of remoxipride necessary to induce catalepsy in rats is markedly higher than that needed to block apomorphine-induced hyperactivity (compared with the equivalent doses for haloperidol and chlorpromazine), which suggests that remoxipride has higher affinity for mesolimbic dopaminergic receptors than for those in striatal areas (Ogren et al. 1990).

Remoxipride appeared to be a valuable addition to the antipsychotic armamentarium and gained approval for clinical use in 15 countries. Unfortunately, several deaths secondary to aplastic anemia in remoxipride-treated patients were recently reported in Europe and necessitated its withdrawal from clinical use. Therefore, it is currently unlikely that remoxipride will be approved in the United States. This experience is an example of the uncertainties that revolve around the development of new medications and underscores the necessity for careful and complete clinical evaluation of all novel antipsychotic medications.

Strategies for Drug Development

Despite the promise of these new antipsychotic drugs, they do not represent "ideal" treatments. Most patients treated with these drugs will continue to display some behavioral manifestations of their illness while enduring various side effects (Malhotra et al. 1993). It is telling that clozapine, the prototype for many of these drugs, is not considered to be a "cure" for schizophrenia and is still associated with a diverse side-effect profile that includes agranulocytosis. It is hoped that these new agents will prove to be as effective as clozapine without many of its concomitant side effects. Even so, it is clear that new drug strategies are still needed to continue the progress in fighting this devastating illness. What are some potential avenues of investigation for these new strategies?

Hyperdopaminergic Agents

One idea that has generated considerable interest stems from a reformulation of the original dopamine hypothesis of schizophrenia. Several studies have suggested that, in fact, hypodopaminergic function in cortical areas is involved in the pathophysiology of schizophrenia that leads to or is correlated with a hyperdopaminergic state within subcortical structures (Davis et al. 1991). In this model, typical neuroleptics would act on the subcortical hyperdopaminergic state to reduce the positive symptoms of the illness while exacerbating preexisting cortical dysfunction and, perhaps, negative symptoms. If this is the case, medications that increase cortical dopaminergic function while depressing subcortical dopaminergic activity might more effectively treat both symptom complexes of schizophrenia. Several studies have attempted to achieve this by augmenting typical neuroleptic treatment with dopamine agonists such as amphetamine or methylphenidate (M. D. Carpenter et al. 1992; Goldberg et al. 1991). Another approach involves administration of agents such as preclamol, a partial dopamine agonist and potent dopamine autoreceptor agonist, in an attempt to reduce psychotic symptoms (Tamminga et al. 1992). These efforts suggest that this strategy may be important in antipsychotic efficacy, and further work may propose future directions for drug development.

D_4 Antagonists

Another area of active investigation for drug developers is the role of non-D_2-dopaminergic receptors in schizophrenia and antipsychotic drug efficacy. In particular, the D_4 receptor has attracted interest with the initial finding that clozapine is a potent D_4-receptor antagonist (Van Tol et al. 1991). Subsequent postmortem work demonstrated significantly increased density of D_4 receptors in brains of patients with schizophrenia (Seeman et al. 1993). New compounds specifically for the D_4 receptor are under investigation, and future work defining these compounds' therapeutic efficacy will be of enormous interest to drug developers.

Noradrenergic Agents

Another avenue for research into antipsychotic drug efficacy is the role of the noradrenergic system. A potentially important aspect of clozapine's mechanism of action is its remarkable effect on noradrenergic turnover. Breier et al. (1994) demonstrated significant increases in plasma norepinephrine levels with clozapine, in contrast to haloperidol, that correlated with clinical response. In addition, Litman et al. (1993) reported that an α_2 antagonist, idazoxan, augments therapeutic response to fluphenazine in patients with chronic schizophrenia. These data suggest that the noradrenergic system may be important in achieving therapeutic efficacy. New agents focused on this neurotransmitter system may be of interest in the future.

Glutamatergic Agents

The glutamatergic system has also been implicated in the pathophysiology of schizophrenia. Glutamate, the most abundant excitatory neurotransmitter in the brain, plays a critical role in perception, information processing, and memory—functions impaired in schizophrenia (Javitt and Zukin 1990). In addition, phencyclidine, a well-known psychotogenic drug, produces its effects via interference with the glutamatergic *N*-methyl-D-aspartate (NMDA) receptor (Javitt and Zukin 1991). Decreased corticolimbic glutamate activity has therefore been hypothesized to be involved in the pathophysiology of schizophrenia, and compounds that augment glutamatergic activity may be important for future treatment strategies. To test this theory, several investigators administered glycine, an allosteric modulator of the NMDA receptor, to patients with schizophrenia as monotherapy or in conjunction with traditional neuroleptics. In an open trial, Waziri (1988) reported neuroleptic dose reductions in 4 of 11 patients treated with glycine, whereas Zukin et al. (1993) reported modest improvement in psychotic symptoms in patients treated with high oral doses of glycine. Treatment with glycine is hampered by its relative impermeability through the blood-brain barrier. To counter this, Rosse et al. (1991) administered milacemide, a "prodrug" of glycine that crosses the blood-brain barrier and is then converted to glycine, to 4 patients. Although they reported no overall antipsychotic efficacy, 1 of the 4 patients experienced marked reductions in negative symptom ratings with milacemide treatment. Future work in drug development may attempt to utilize these data to devise new compounds that can augment NMDA activity and reduce psychotic symptoms.

G-Protein Effectors

Another active area of investigation is G-protein research. G proteins are ubiquitous and critical for a variety of cell functions (Manji 1992). Dopamine receptors are linked to G proteins, and dysfunction in this link has been found in brains of patients with schizophrenia (Seeman et al. 1989). As data continue to accumulate suggesting that the site of antipsychotic efficacy is "downstream" from the receptors located on cell membranes, it may be reasonable to target the G proteins for psychopharmacological investigations. Development of drugs that act directly on specific G proteins is probably several years away; however, available techniques such as "antisense" deoxyribonucleic acid (DNA) can affect protein synthesis (Zhang and Creese 1993). If specific abnormalities can be identified in G-protein function in schizophrenia, drug developers may be able to use these techniques to design increasingly effective treatments.

Conclusion

As the revolution in neuroscience continues, new hypotheses about the pathophysiology of schizophrenia and the mechanism of action of antipsychotic drugs have led to fundamental changes in drug development. It is hoped that the medications closest to approval for general availability will be more efficacious and produce less serious side effects than current medications. By designing drugs with specific properties, drug developers hope to achieve the therapeutic profile of clozapine and extend its benefits to patients unable to tolerate clozapine. These novel antipsychotics may be the treatments of choice for thousands of patients with schizophrenia, and clinicians must be cognizant of patients' relative strengths and weaknesses when devising treatment strategies. In the future, it is reasonable to foresee the introduction of medications unrelated to currently available drugs as neuroscientists develop and test new hypotheses about schizophrenia.

References

Axelsson R, Nilsson A, Christensson E, et al: Effects of amperozide in schizophrenia: an open study of a potent $5HT_2$ receptor antagonist. Psychopharmacology 104:287–292, 1991

Borison RL, Pathiraja AP, Diamond BI: Risperidone: clinical safety and efficacy in schizophrenia. Psychopharmacol Bull 28:213–218, 1992

Breier A, Schreiber JL, Dyer J, et al: National Institute of Mental Health longitudinal study of chronic schizophrenia: prognosis and prediction of outcome. Arch Gen Psychiatry 48:239–246, 1991

Breier A, Buchanan RW, Irish D, et al: Clozapine treatment of outpatients with schizophrenia: outcome and long-term response patterns. Hosp Community Psychiatry 44:1145–1149, 1993

Breier A, Buchanan RW, Waltrip II RW, et al: The effect of clozapine on plasma norepinephrine: relationship to clinical efficacy. Neuropsychopharmacology 10:1–7, 1994

Carpenter MD, Winsberg BG, Camus LA: Methylphenidate augmentation therapy in schizophrenia. J Clin Psychopharmacol 12:273–275, 1992

Carpenter WT, Conley RR, Buchanan RW, et al: Patient response and resource management: another view of clozapine treatment of schizophrenia. Am J Psychiatry 152:827–832, 1995

Chiodo LA, Bunney BD: Typical and atypical neuroleptics differential effects of chronic administration on the activity of A9 and A10 midbrain dopaminergic neurons. J Neurosci 3:1607–1619, 1983

Chouinard G: Early phase II clinical trial of remoxipride in treatment of schizophrenia with measurements of prolactin and neuroleptic activity. J Clin Psychopharmacol 3:159–164, 1987

Chouinard G: A placebo-controlled clinical trial of remoxipride and chlorpromazine in newly admitted schizophrenic patients with acute exacerbation. Acta Psychiatr Scand 82 (suppl 358):11–119, 1990

Chouinard G, Jones G, Remington G, et al: A Canadian multicenter placebo-controlled study of fixed doses of risperidone and haloperidol in the treatment of chronic schizophrenic patients. J Clin Psychopharmacol 13:25–40, 1993

Christensson EG, Bjork A: Amperozide: a new pharmacological approach in the treatment of schizophrenia. Pharmacol Toxicol (suppl 1):5–7, 1990

Christensson EG, Gustafsson B: Amperozide, a novel psychotropic compound with specific effect on limbic brain areas (abstract). Acta Physiol Scand 124 (suppl 542):281, 1985

Davis KL, Kahn RS, Ko G, et al: Dopamine in schizophrenia: a review and reconceptualization. Am J Psychiatry 148:1474–1486, 1991

Fabre L, Slotnick V, Jones V, et al: ICI 204.636, a novel atypical antipsychotic: early indications for safety and efficacy in man, in Abstracts of the 17th Congress of CINP, Vol 2. Kyoto, Japan, 1990

Fenton WS, McGlashan TH: Antecedents, symptom progression and long-term outcome of the deficit syndrome in schizophrenia. Am J Psychiatry 151:351–356, 1994

Fuller RW, Snoddy HD: Neuroendocrine evidence for antagonism of serotonin and dopamine receptors by olanzapine (LY170053), an antipsychotic drug candidate. Res Commun Chem Pathol Pharmacol 77:87–93, 1992

Goldberg TE, Bigelow LB, Weinberger DR, et al: Cognitive and behavioral effects of the coadministration of dextroamphetamine and haloperidol in schizophrenia. Am J Psychiatry 148:78–84, 1991

Janssen PA, Niemegeers CJ, Awouters F, et al: Pharmacology of risperidone (R 64 766), a new antipsychotic with serotonin-S2 and dopamine-D2 antagonistic properties. J Pharmacol Exp Ther 244:685–693, 1988

Javitt DC, Zukin SR: The role of excitatory amino acids in neuropsychiatric illness. J Neuropsychiatry Clin Neurosci 2:44–52, 1990

Javitt DC, Zukin SR: Recent advances in the phencyclidine model of schizophrenia. Am J Psychiatry 148:1301–1308, 1991

Kane J, Honigfeld G, Singer J, et al: Clozapine for the treatment-resistant schizophrenic: a double-blind comparison with chlorpromazine. Arch Gen Psychiatry 45:789–796, 1988

Lewander T, Westerbergh SE, Morrison D: Clinical profile of remoxipride—a combined analysis of a comparative double-blind multicenter trial programme. Acta Psychiatr Scand 82 (suppl 358):92–98, 1990

Litman RE, Hong WW, Weissman EM, et al: Idazoxan, an α_2 antagonist, augments fluphenazine response in schizophrenic patients: a pilot study. J Clin Psychopharmacol 13:264–267, 1993

Malhotra AK, Litman RE, Pickar D: Adverse effects of antipsychotic drugs. Drug Saf 9:429–436, 1993

Malick JB, Migler BM, Salama AI: ICI 204.636: a new and novel atypical antipsychotic drug (abstract). Schizophr Res 3:46, 1990

Manji HK: G proteins: implications for psychiatry. Am J Psychiatry 149:746–760, 1992

Meltzer HY: Clozapine: mechanism of action in relation to its clinical advantages, in Recent Advances in Schizophrenia. Edited by Kales A, Stefanis CN, Talbott J. New York, Springer-Verlag, 1990, pp 237–256

Meltzer HY, Zhang Y, Stockmeier CA: Effect of amperozide on rat cortical $5HT_2$ and striatal and limbic dopamine D_2 receptor occupancy: implication for antipsychotic action. Eur J Pharmacol 216:67–71, 1992

Mertens C, De Wilde J, Dierick M, et al: Clinical trials of amperozide in schizophrenia (abstract). Excerpta Medica International Congress Series VIIth World Congress of Psychiatry 899:502, 1989

Moore NA, Tye NC, Axton MS, et al: The behavioral pharmacology of olanzapine, a novel "atypical" antipsychotic agent. J Pharmacol Exp Ther 262:545–551, 1992

Ogren SO, Florvall L, Hall H, et al: Neuropharmacological and behavioral properties of remoxipride in the rat. Acta Psychiatr Scand 82 (suppl 358):21–26, 1990

Overall JE, Gorham DR: The Brief Psychiatric Rating Sale. Psychol Rep 10:799–812, 1962

Pickar D, Owen RR, Litman RE, et al: Clinical and biologic response to clozapine in patients with schizophrenia: crossover comparison with fluphenazine. Arch Gen Psychiatry 49:345–353, 1992

Rosse RB, Schwartz BL, Davis RE, et al: An NMDA intervention strategy in schizophrenia with "low dose" milacemide. Clin Neuropharmacol 14:268–272, 1991

Roy A: Suicide in chronic schizophrenia. Br J Psychiatry 141:171–177, 1982

Seeman P, Niznik HB, Guan HC, et al: Link between D_1 and D_2 dopamine receptors is reduced in schizophrenia and Huntington diseased brain. Proc Natl Acad Sci U S A 86:10156–10160, 1989

Seeman P, Guan HC, Van Tol HHM: Dopamine D_4 receptors elevated in schizophrenia. Nature 365:441–446, 1993

Skarsfeldt T, Perregaard J: Sertindole, a new neuroleptic with extreme selectivity on A10 versus A9 dopaminergic neurons in the rat. Eur J Pharmacol 182:613–614, 1990

Svartengren J, Simonsson P: Receptor binding properties of amperozide. Pharmacol Toxicol 66 (suppl 1):8–11, 1990

Tamminga CA, Cascella NG, Lahti RA, et al: Pharmacologic properties of (-)-3ppp (preclamol) in man. J Neural Transm Gen Sect 88:165–175, 1992

Tollefson GD, Beasley CM, Tran PV, et al: Olanzapine: a novel antipsychotic with a broad spectrum profile. Paper presented at the 49th annual meeting of the Society of Biological Psychiatry, Philadelphia, PA, May 1994

Van Tol HHM, Bunzow JR, Guan HC, et al: Cloning of the gene for a human dopamine D_4 receptor with high affinity for the antipsychotic clozapine. Nature 350:610–614, 1991

Wadworth AN, Heel RC: Remoxipride: a review of its pharmacodynamic and pharmacokinetic properties and therapeutic potential in schizophrenia. Drugs 40:863–879, 1990

Waziri R: Glycine therapy of schizophrenia. Biol Psychiatry 23:210–211, 1988

Zhang M, Creese I: Antisense oligodeoxynucleotide reduces brain dopamine D_2 receptors: behavioral correlates. Neurosci Lett 161:223–226, 1993

Zukin SR, Javitt DC, Nussenzveig IZ, et al: NMDA receptor stimulation in schizophrenia. Paper presented at the 146th annual meeting of the American Psychiatric Association, San Francisco, CA, May 22–27, 1993

CHAPTER 4

New Neuroleptics and Experimental Antipsychotics: Future Roles

Adrienne C. Lahti, M.D.
Robert A. Lahti, Ph.D.
Carol A. Tamminga, M.D.

The need for new drugs to treat schizophrenia clearly exists. Available neuroleptics often incompletely treat psychotic symptoms and produce serious side effects. Studies with clozapine have demonstrated that new treatments can provide additional antipsychotic efficacy (Kane et al. 1988). Currently available antipsychotic drugs treat some patients and some symptoms successfully but leave many patients with schizophrenia partially or extensively untreated. Some symptom complexes are characteristically inadequately treated by neuroleptics, such as social and cognitive deficits; negative symptoms can even worsen with neuroleptics (Lader 1993). Moreover, side effects of current neuroleptics are burdensome and sometimes serious. The long-lasting neuroleptic-induced motor side effect of tardive dyskinesia is especially limiting.

Which are the viable antipsychotic strategies to pursue now and into the twenty-first century? What are the main candidate drugs in those areas? These major questions are addressed in this chapter. Antipsychotic drug development strategies can be organized into several main groups:

1. Refined clozapine-like strategies
2. Novel antidopaminergic approaches
3. Experimental strategies based on speculative hypotheses of psychosis/schizophrenia
4. More serendipity

We review in detail the first three of the above categories. The last item deserves separate mention. Serendipity has contributed pivotally to many advances in somatic treatments in psychiatry. Pathophysiology is unknown for all of the major psychiatric diseases, including schizophrenia. Without known pathophysiology to direct drug discovery, informed and creative serendipity becomes important. A clue to successful antidepressant treatment came with the observation of antidepressant benefit with isoniazid during tuberculosis treatment (Crane 1959; Kline 1958). The direction of antipsychotic treatment was fixed for a half-century by the observation of selective antipsychotic activity of a known sedative (Delay and Deniker 1952). Other examples, such as depression and anxiety disorders, also support the importance of critical clinical observation in new drug development. Recognizing the role of serendipity does not diminish the ultimate goal of attempting rational strategies for new drug development. Rational therapies can be developed on the basis of already successful strategies but not yet on pathophysiology.

Refined Clozapine-like Strategies

Clozapine is a dibenzodiazepine. It has a very broad receptor affinity profile, demonstrating measurable affinity for the D_1, D_2, D_3, D_4, α_1, α_2, 5-HT_2, 5-HT_{1a}, H_1, and nicotinic and muscarinic cholinergic receptors. This complex receptor profile makes it difficult to link receptor characteristics with clinical actions. Clozapine has a low but measurable affinity for the striatal D_2 receptor and, in vivo, appears to preferentially selectively influence limbic dopamine (DA) receptors. Clozapine has very high affinity for the D_4 receptor relative to the D_2 receptor. Based on these neurochemical characteristics of clozapine, several new directions are being pursued in therapeutics.

Broad Receptor Blockade

Clozapine has relatively high and balanced affinity for a broad range of monoaminergic, cholinergic, and histaminergic receptors, which are present in dorsal and ventral striatum and cortex (Coward 1992). Rat and mouse experiments indicate that several of these receptors interact to produce striatal functions in the face of inhibited DA transmission and, presumably, therefore, interact with DA in normal striatal function (Carlsson et al. 1991). It would be plausible to imagine that clozapine has its unique properties because of these combined antagonist receptor actions. One might hypothesize, based on this rationale, that improved antipsychotic action will derive from a broad, balanced receptor antagonism in striatum.

Several new drugs being studied appear to fit this category. Olanzapine, a thienobenzodiazepine, has a receptor-affinity profile nearly as broad as that of clozapine (Moore 1992) (Table 4–1). Because it lacks nicotinic cholinergic antagonism, some of clozapine's side effects like sialorrhea may be avoided. Olanzapine also shows a "limbic selectivity" in its effects on neuronal populations and on animal behaviors. In its earliest controlled clinical studies, olanzapine demonstrated potent antipsychotic action in schizophrenia with a low level of parkinsonism and akathisia (Harrison et al. 1994).

Selective Combinations of Receptor Blockade

Several different studies have consistently supported the role of D_2-family blockade in the mechanism of action of antipsychotic drugs (Creese et al. 1976; Kebabian and Calne 1979; Peroutka and Snyder 1980; Seeman et al. 1976; Snyder et al. 1975). Whether an additional neurochemical action might improve or extend that action has often been suggested but never fully supported. Indeed, the many studies involving "add-on" treatments for schizophrenia support the general validity of this approach. Clinical scientists have attempted to add lithium (Biederman et al. 1979; Hirschowitz et al. 1980; Small et al. 1975), antidepressants (Prusoff et al. 1979; Siris et al. 1978, 1985; Waehrens and Gerlach 1980),

Table 4–1. Binding profile of various compounds

Compound	K_i (nM) at various receptors										
	D_1	D_2	D_3[a]	D_4[a]	5-HT_2	5-HT_{1a}	5-HT_{1c}[a]	Muscarinic	α_1	α_2	Sigma
Haloperidol	25	1	6	3	25	3,080	4,170	1,475	46	360	17
Chlorpromazine		2	7	16	1.5	—	5	—	—	—	—
Clozapine	85	82[b]	609	29	1.4	120	11	2	8.5	80.5	1,600
Remoxipride		132[b]	4,053	> 5,000	5,112	—	5,120	—	—	—	—
Olanzapine	31	11[b]	—	27	5	> 5,000	23	2	19	228	—
Sertindole	28	1.5[b]	—	2.8	0.4	2,600	—	2,500	3.4	350	73
Risperidone	534	3.1	—	—	0.16	253	—	< 5	0.8	7.5	—
Seroquel[c]	1,243	329[b]	—	—	148	720	—	> 10,000	90	270	—

Note. — = not available.
[a]Cloned receptor preparations. [b]Mesolimbic selective. [c]IC_{50} (nM) values.

benzodiazepines (Csernansky et al. 1988; Douyon et al. 1989; Wolkowitz et al. 1988), and other antipsychotic drugs to neuroleptic drugs to extend their action in treating schizophrenia. Although many of these reports have claimed positive therapeutic actions, none has demonstrated that the add-on compound actually enhanced the primary antipsychotic action of the neuroleptic.

Based on the observation that ritanserin, a potent 5-HT_2 antagonist, appeared to enhance the effects of haloperidol and reduce motor side effects (Bersani et al. 1986; Gelders et al. 1986), the idea to develop an enhanced neuroleptic drug with combined D_2/5-HT_2 action began (Janssen et al. 1988; Leysen et al. 1988). Considerable evidence supports the logic that dopaminergic and serotonergic systems in the mammalian central nervous system (CNS) functionally interact (Herve et al. 1981; Nicolaou et al. 1979; Rasmussen and Aghajanian 1988) and may provide an enhanced antipsychotic effect (Claghorn et al. 1987; Kane et al. 1988; Meltzer 1989; Meltzer et al. 1990). Based on this rationale, risperidone was developed (Borison et al. 1992; Chouinard et al. 1993; Marder 1992). Risperidone has potent D_2 and 5-HT_2 antagonist activities and is now marketed as an antipsychotic drug, the first to be approved since clozapine. It appears to have a motor side-effect advantage in lower dose ranges, with a diminished advantage at higher doses. Whether it will have additional advantages or antipsychotic effect in clinical application remains to be discovered. Several additional drugs being developed exemplify the strategy of D_2/5-HT_2 action. These include sertindole and seroquel. Sertindole is an imidazolidinone with at least moderate affinity for the D_1, D_2, 5-HT_2, and α_1 receptors and with a dose-related functional limbic selectivity (Skarsfeldt and Perregaard 1990). At a dose of 20 mg/day, it is effective in treating schizophrenia, well tolerated, and associated with a very low incidence of extrapyramidal side effects (EPS) (Martin et al. 1994). Seroquel, a dibenzothiazepine, has high affinity for 5-HT_2 receptors as well as for the D_2, α_2, α_1, and H_1 receptors. In an open trial pilot study of inpatients with acute psychotic symptoms, it was found to be well tolerated and effective, with few EPS (Fabre 1993).

Clozapine has the almost unique characteristic among neuroleptics of a balanced D_1 and D_2 antagonism. The role of D_1 antagonism in schizophrenia is poorly understood. Although a study with the selective D_1 antagonist SCH 39166 has been concluded, outcome has not yet been reported. Moreover, whether D_1 antagonism will enhance D_2 blockade–mediated antipsychotic action is an open and interesting question. One of the newest putative antipsychotic drugs—SDZ DOD 647—has, among other properties, the balanced D_1/D_2 antagonism of clozapine, to test this strategy. Several similar drugs are being developed as antipsychotics.

Potent α_2 antagonism is also one of clozapine's prominent characteristics. A trial of α_2 blockade in schizophrenia is further supported by several data that norepinephrine (NE) is elevated in schizophrenia. The transmitter has been shown to be increased in the cerebrospinal fluid (CSF) of patients with schizophrenia (Gattaz et al. 1983; Gomes et al. 1980; Kemali et al. 1982; Lake et al. 1980) and in some brain areas postmortem (Bird et al. 1979; Crow et al. 1979; Farley et al. 1978; Kleinman et al. 1979). Idazoxan, an α_2 antagonist, has been tested for its ability to enhance the antipsychotic action of a typical neuroleptic such as haloperidol. Initial data are encouraging (Litman et al. 1993). Several of the new antipsychotic drugs incorporate this feature.

Low D_2 Receptor Affinity

Clozapine has a low affinity for the D_2 receptor. Its inhibition constant (K_i) at the cloned D_2 receptor is 82 nM, at the D_3 is 609 nM, and at the D_4 is 29 nM. When tested using in vivo techniques, not only does this affinity remain low, but also the distribution of the clozapine effect on DA neurons (Bunney 1984) and DA projection field (see Deutch et al. 1991 for review) appears predominantly in the "limbic" DA projection fields, including nucleus accumbens shell, medial prefrontal cortex, and cingulate. Chronic administration of clozapine affects only the ventral tegmental area (VTA) A10 DA neurons (i.e., those neurons whose cell bodies are in the VTA and project to limbic and neocortical areas), causing depolarization blockade. This localized antidopaminergic action might account for the reduced motor side effects with clozapine compared with other neuroleptics and, possibly, its unique antipsychotic action. Hence, clinicians have become interested in drugs with these pharmacological characteristics. Remoxipride, a 6-methoxy benzamide, exhibits low affinity for the D_2 receptor and moderate sigma affinity at clinical doses. Like clozapine, it has been shown to be limbic selective (Kohler et al. 1990). Human positron-emission tomography (PET) occupancy studies suggest that therapeutic doses produce at 50%–70% striatal D_2-receptor occupancy, compared with 80%–90% for haloperidol (Farde and von Bahr 1990). Remoxipride is effective in the treatment of schizophrenia and shows a low incidence of EPS and little sedation (Lewander et al. 1990). In a double-blind, haloperidol-controlled, preliminary study, remoxipride produced a response rate in a treatment-resistant schizophrenic population similar to that of clozapine (Conley and Tamminga 1994). Although remoxipride development for general clinical use has been interrupted because of its untoward and often lethal aplastic anemia side effect, attention to its pharmacological and clinical characteristics remains important.

Relatively High D_4 Receptor Affinity

Clozapine has a relatively high affinity for the D_4 receptor compared with its affinity for the D_2 receptor. This suggests the possible importance of D_4-receptor antagonism in antipsychotic treatments. The rationale for D_4-receptor antagonism in schizophrenia has now extended beyond the clozapine rationale (R. A. Lahti et al. 1993; Seeman et al. 1993; Van Tol et al. 1991). This strategy is discussed in the subsection later in this chapter, "Selective D_4- or D_3-Receptor Blockade."

Novel Antidopaminergic Approaches

Because reduction in DA-mediated neuronal transmission through D_2-receptor blockade has already been demonstrated to provide selective antipsychotic activity, perhaps other techniques to diminish dopaminergic transmission might also be antipsychotic. Several strategies to accomplish this are already available (Table 4–2), and some are being tested.

Partial Dopamine Agonists

Partial DA agonists have full affinity for the DA receptor but only partial intrinsic activity (compared with the endogenous ligand). Affinity is a measure of the strength with which a receptor binds a drug; intrinsic activity is a measure of the effectiveness of that drug in stimulating the receptor (Kenakin 1993). The degree of

Table 4–2. Strategies for antipsychotic drug development

Broad monoaminergic receptor blockade (e.g., clozapine)
5-HT_2/D_2-family receptor blockade (e.g., risperidone)
Selective D_2-family receptor blockade (e.g., remoxipride)
D_1/D_2-family receptor blockade (e.g., SDZ DOD 647)
Other transmitter blockade combinations (e.g., sertindole, olanzapine)
Partial dopamine agonists (e.g., (-)-3PPP)
Cotransmitter modulation (e.g., CP 99994)
Selective D_4- or D_3-receptor blockade (e.g., UH232)
Anatomically selective D_2 antagonists (e.g., savoxepin)

intrinsic activity is unique to each partial agonist and can be expressed as a percentage of the activation produced by the full agonist (DA, in this instance) in a given paradigm (Figure 4–1). Partial agonists can act as functional agonists under conditions of low transmitter concentration or as functional antagonists under conditions of high endogenous transmitter release (because of dilution by a lower intrinsic activity agonist). The use of partial DA agonists in the treatment of schizophrenia is based on their preferential affinity for, and agonist activity at, the DA autoreceptor. The autoreceptor is located on the DA neuron itself and functions to decrease DA synthesis and release (reviewed in Tamminga et al. 1986a). Both D_2 and D_3 subtypes are autoreceptors. The somatodendritic autoreceptors modulate cell firing, and the terminal autoreceptors modulate neurotransmitter synthesis and release. Activation of the DA autoreceptor reduces DA synthesis, release from presynaptic terminals, and firing of the cell. This would theoretically result in reduced DA-mediated neural transmission and, thus, exert a neuroleptic-like effect in psychotic illness. A therapeutic window could be a result of this dual action of the partial DA agonist: at lower concentrations, a partial agonist will bind to the autoreceptor and putatively have a neuroleptic-like effect; at higher concentrations, it will bind to the DA-rich postsynaptic receptor and putatively have a postsynaptic agonist-like effect.

Apomorphine has been reported to decrease psychotic symptoms in patients with schizophrenia (Corsini et al. 1977, 1981; Jeste et al. 1983; Tamminga et al. 1978); however, all studies have not consistently concurred (Ferrier et al. 1984; Levy et al. 1984). Other

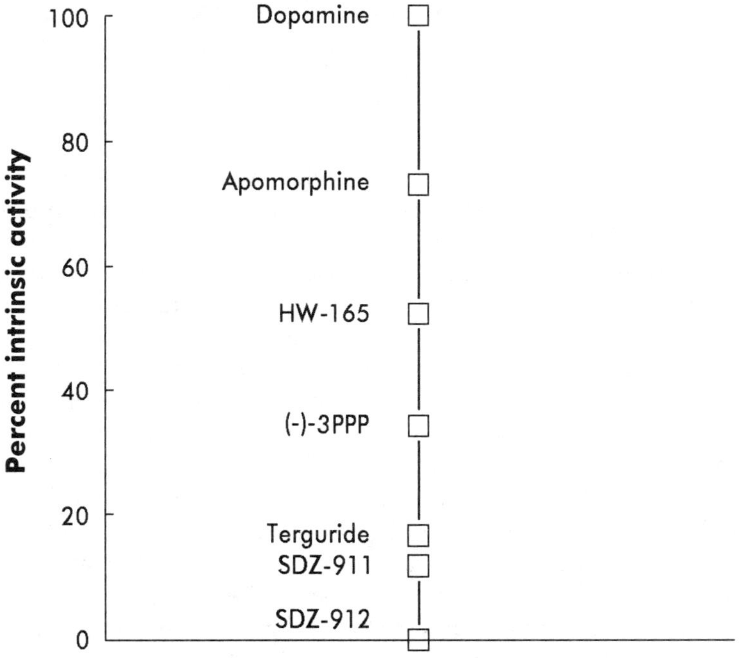

Figure 4–1. The rank order intrinsic activity of dopamine agonists and partial agonists as determined using receptor state binding affinity ratios.

full DA agonists like bromocriptine, CF 25397, and piribedil in a low dose range failed to show an antipsychotic action (Brambilla et al. 1983; Meltzer 1980; Tamminga and Schaffer 1979). N-propylnorapomorphine (NPA), a full DA agonist and structural analogue of apomorphine, showed an acute antipsychotic action, but repeated administration produced tolerance to this effect (Tamminga et al. 1986a). Partial DA agonists provide a new opportunity to test this strategy. Knowledge about different compounds with varying levels of intrinsic activity would reveal which level of this activity produces the most favorable antipsychotic action, if any. Several partial or full DA agonists are currently being tested for the treatment of schizophrenia: (-)-3PPP (preclamol), SND 919 (premipexole), PD 143188, SDZ-HDC 912 (Naber 1991; Potkin et al. 1993), PD 128483, B-HT 920 (tolipexole)

(Ohmori et al. 1993; Wiedemann et al. 1992), EMD 49980 (roxindole) (Wetzel and Benkert 1993; Wiedemann et al. 1990, 1992), OPC-4392 (Gerbaldo et al. 1988), and terguride (Olbrich and Schanz 1988). These agonists have different intrinsic activities at the cloned D_2 receptor (Figure 4–1).

(-)-3PPP is a partial DA agonist with approximately 35% intrinsic activity at the expressed D_2 receptor. In animal experiments, it acts preferentially in limbic regions as an agonist. (-)-3PPP reduces open field exploratory behavior in rats following injection into nucleus accumbens, but not into dorsal striatum, and affects DA turnover in the nucleus accumbens but not in dorsal striatum (L. Svensson and Ahlenius 1983). At higher doses, it acts as a postsynaptic D_2 agonist, mimicking the action of haloperidol on globus pallidus neuronal firing (Bergstrom et al. 1986). This might be a result of its low level of intrinsic activity at the DA receptor, as well as the receptor environment. On the other hand, (-)-3PPP does not exhibit affinities for α_1, α_2, β, 5-HT_2, or 5-HT_{1a} receptors. This otherwise "clean" profile makes (-)-3PPP an ideal candidate to test the hypothesis of partial DA agonist therapy in schizophrenia. Actively psychotic, drug-free volunteers with schizophrenia have already received (-)-3PPP or placebo in single rising doses (between 1 and 40 mg im) to achieve target plasma levels of 200–500 pmol/ml (an estimated active plasma level range from preclinical studies) (Tamminga et al. 1992b). Based on preliminary efficacy estimates, some antipsychotic activity was seen. Several subjects showed some level of an acute antipsychotic action after the higher doses. Based on this study, an efficacy trial of (-)-3PPP is being conducted in a crossover, fixed-dose, placebo-controlled design.

Partial DA agonists might also competitively dilute the potency with which a DA antagonist can produce motor side effects without having its own psychotomimetic effect. Consistent with this is the report that schizophrenic patients with parkinsonism who were treated with terguride concurrent with their neuroleptic showed a reduction in the motor side effect (Filip et al. 1992). In a supportive preclinical study, K. Svensson and Carlsson (1993) showed that haloperidol induced catalepsy and was antagonized by (-)-3PPP. Studies in humans have begun to test whether (-)-3PPP will be an effective adjunct medication to treat haloperidol-induced akathisia and parkinsonism.

B-HT 920 (Ohmori et al. 1993), EMD 49980 (Wiedemann et al. 1992), and SDZ-HDC 912 (Naber 1991; Potkin et al. 1993) have been tested in patients with schizophrenia with mixed results. High intrinsic activity agonists appear to reduce negative, but not positive, symptoms. The lowest intrinsic activity agonist—SDZ-HDC 912—improved positive symptoms but also produced motor side effects. The optimal intrinsic activity, if one exists, has not yet been found.

Cotransmitter Modulation

Many DA-containing neurons also contain a peptide that often behaves like a neuromodulator. These peptides are presumably cosecreted with DA and then modulate the activity of the DA neuron itself, the impact of the released transmitter (DA) on the postsynaptic neuron, or (independently) the activity of the postsynaptic neuron. Two peptides frequently colocalized with DA are cholecystokinin (CCK), an eight amino acid peptide, and neurotensin (NT), a tridecapeptide. Clinical application of peptide therapies has been slow because peptide to CNS access is difficult across the blood-brain barrier, the ability of peptides to pass into CNS tissue is very low, and rapid degradation by plasma and tissue peptidase occurs. Nonpeptidergic agonists and antagonists of these receptors must be available for clinical testing.

CCK-8 is a peptidergic transmitter, and some of its neurochemical features suggest potential interest for schizophrenia—for example, its cortical localization (Beinfeld et al. 1981) and colocalization with DA in certain mesencephalic DA-containing neurons, particularly in the A10 regions (Hokfelt et al. 1980). Despite promising preclinical data in animal models (Crawley and Vanderhaegen 1985), the controlled clinical experiments have been uniformly negative (Hommer et al. 1984; Lotstra et al. 1984; Tamminga et al. 1986b). One explanation is that CCK-8 fails to enter the mammalian brain with systemic administration. Thus, the hypothesis that CCK-8 will reduce psychosis in schizophrenia has not yet been effectively tested because of the problem of effective delivery. One way to solve the drug delivery problem is to develop nonpeptide agonists and antagonists for the receptor or to target the modulation of nonreceptor sites in the biosynthetic pathways such as cell-surface receptors or transcription regulatory protein. A number of pharmaceutical manufacturers are developing such candidates.

A growing body of evidence has implicated NT in the pathophysiology of schizophrenia as well as in the mechanism of action of antipsychotic drugs. In animals, centrally applied NT produces effects similar to exogenously administered antipsychotic drugs such as increase in DA turnover, decrease in conditioned avoidance response, antagonism of amphetamine-induced locomotor activity, and induction of hypothermia (see Stowe and Nemeroff 1993 for review). NT concentration in the CSF is decreased in drug-free patients with schizophrenia (Garver et al. 1991; Lindstrom et al. 1988; Widerlov et al. 1982) and increased after administration of antipsychotic drugs (Garver et al. 1991; Widerlov et al. 1982). NT is increased in the nucleus accumbens and striatum of postmortem schizophrenic brains (Nemeroff et al. 1983). Finally, acute and chronic administration of typical antipsychotic drugs increases NT concentrations in the nucleus accumbens and caudate (Frey et al. 1988; Govoni et al. 1980; Kilts et al. 1988), whereas the atypical antipsychotic drug clozapine increases NT only in the nucleus accumbens (Kilts et al. 1988). Speculatively, this could account for the difference between typical and atypical antipsychotics. The availability of the NT-cloned receptor (Tanaka et al. 1990) may foster the development of nonpeptidergic NT-receptor agonists for the treatment of schizophrenia.

CP 99994 is a nonpeptide substance P antagonist being studied in patients with schizophrenia. Substance P is an undecapeptide of the tachykinin family. It acts both as a neurotransmitter and a neuromodulator in various body systems. Several indirect lines of evidence implicate substance P in the pathophysiology of schizophrenia. Substance P immunoactivity is increased in the hippocampus of postmortem schizophrenic brains compared with control brains (Roberts et al. 1983). Mesocortical DA neuronal activation by footshock stress is blocked by substance P monoclonal antibodies (Bannon et al. 1983). NE is elevated in schizophrenic CSF and brain, and substance P–induced excitation of neurons in the locus coeruleus is reversed by a nonpeptidergic substance P antagonist (McLean et al. 1991). An exploratory, controlled evaluation of the efficacy of CP 99994 is being conducted in schizophrenic patients, but the results are not yet known.

Anatomically Selective D_2 Antagonists

Based on various pharmacological, anatomical, and electrophysiological data, the idea that the areas of the CNS that are involved predominantly with psychotic symptoms are limbic regions (e.g., hippocampus, cingulate, nucleus accumbens, and ventral pallidum) has been proposed and has received considerable support. Postmortem studies have identified morphometric changes in the hippocampus (Bogerts et al. 1985; Falkai and Bogerts 1986); reductions in pyramidal neuronal orientation (Kovelman and Scheibel 1984, Scheibel and Kovelman 1981), cell numbers (Benes 1989; Jeste and Lohr 1989), and nucleus accumbens neuronal density (Pakkenberg 1990); and changes in functional markers of dopaminergic and glutamatergic transmitters (Deakin et al. 1989; Kerwin et al. 1988, 1990). The cingulate cortex also exhibits change (Benes and Bird 1987). Volumetric changes in medial temporal structures have also been reported in structural imaging studies (Bogerts et al. 1990; Breier et al. 1992; Colter et al. 1987; Suddath et al. 1989). A PET study using fluorodeoxyglucose compared schizophrenic patients with healthy subjects and found a significant difference in two brain areas—the anterior cingulate and the hippocampus, two of the three structures forming the Papez circuit—the areas first hypothesized to subserve emotion (Tamminga et al. 1992c). Moreover, in a separate group of patients with schizophrenia, investigators found a correlation between positive symptoms of psychosis and glucose metabolism in the limbic cortex of the right hemisphere. These types of data, which strongly associate positive psychotic symptoms with limbic dysfunction and structural irregularities, support the logic of attempting to target drugs to the hippocampus and cingulate to influence pathological brain areas selectively.

Savoxepine, a tetracyclic derivative, has very potent affinity for the D_2 receptor (K_i = 0.12 nM) and a stated preference for hippocampal versus striatal DA receptors, as suggested by in vivo DA binding studies in rats. Furthermore, the kinetics of DA receptor occupancy demonstrate that this drug has a long duration of DA receptor occupancy, especially in the hippocampus (see Bischoff 1992 for review). In spite of these attractive properties, in clinical studies savoxepine has not shown an advantage over haloperidol in the incidence of EPS (Borison et al. 1993), and preclinical studies have questioned savoxepine's regional selectivity (Cascella et al. 1994).

Selective D_4- or D_3-Receptor Blockade

Knowledge about the structure and localization of brain receptors has increased in the past several years, especially about G protein–coupled receptors. Monoamine receptors of the G protein–coupled type are called *metabotropic.* The recognition site of the receptor is a complex protein, arranged in seven transmembrane spanning segments, an intracellular and extracellular tail, and an important intracellular loop (Figure 4–2). This intracellular loop appears to be one of the sites of coupling between the recognition site and the G protein. The receptor recognition site can undergo

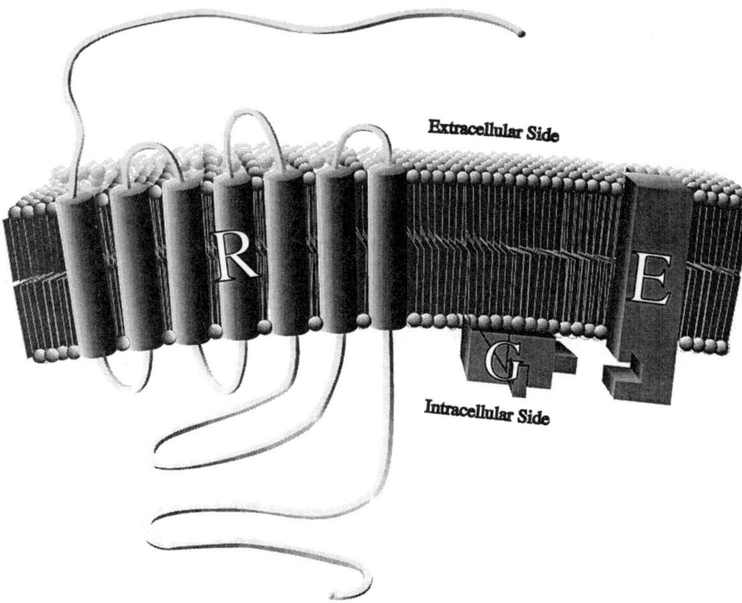

Figure 4–2. G protein–coupled receptor. Receptor consists of an amino acid sequence spanning in and out of the cell membrane (**R**). The binding of a ligand at the receptor produces a cascade of intracellular events, which includes the coupling to G protein (**G**) and the activation/deactivation of an effector protein (**E**).

internalization and degradation with repeated agonist stimulation. Receptors are critically adaptable in an acute and chronic dimension (Caron and Lefkowitz 1993).

Currently, three different DA D_2-family receptors have been cloned and characterized: the DA D_2, D_3, and D_4 receptors. These receptors all interact with the G_i protein complex to inhibit cyclic adenosine monophosphate (cAMP) production. These receptor subtypes can be differentiated genetically, pharmacologically (by different agonist and antagonist), physiologically, and anatomically (by distribution). Their anatomical location in the rat brain has been determined directly, and the location of their neuron's cell bodies has been determined by in situ hybridization studies in which the messenger ribonucleic acid (mRNA) for the receptor is localized. The DA D_2 receptor is densely localized to the striatum, nucleus accumbens, and olfactory tubercles and is present at very low levels in cortical areas. The DA D_3 receptor mRNA is concentrated in the nucleus accumbens and olfactory tubercles and exists in lower levels in the caudate and putamen. The DA D_4 receptor is highly localized to cortical and limbic areas, with lesser amounts in the striatum. Overall, D_3 and D_4 receptors are preferentially localized to limbic areas, whereas D_2 receptors are concentrated in the striatum. Although the quantity of D_2-receptor protein in CNS is relatively high, both the D_3- and D_4-receptor proteins are expressed in far lower quantities, even in their areas of dominant expression.

Research interest in the D_4 receptor has been stimulated by the Seeman et al. (1993) study, which reported a sixfold increase in the density of the D_4 receptors in postmortem schizophrenic brain tissue compared with healthy tissue. Furthermore, it has been recently reported that the D_4 receptor demonstrates a hypervariable repeat region at the level of the third intracytoplasmic loop, the loop putatively responsible for some aspects of G-protein coupling (Van Tol et al. 1992). Although the functional significance of this is not entirely clear, it is possible that D_4 variants will couple to G proteins differently or have distinct pharmacologies. Whether a certain repeat variant might be correlated with drug responsiveness or the expression of schizophrenia is an important question that remains to be answered (Kennedy et al. 1994).

The unique localization of the D_3 receptor to the limbic brain areas makes it an interesting receptor in schizophrenia. Theoretically, a selective D_3 antagonist might demonstrate antipsychotic activity without motor or neuroendocrine side effects because no D_3 receptors have been detected in the pituitary gland. UH232 and AJ76, two putative autoreceptor selective agents (K. Svensson and Carlsson 1993), exhibit preferential affinity at the D_3 receptor. UH232, the most selective D_3 agonist, is currently being tested in patients with schizophrenia.

The D_2 family of DA receptors is all cloned. Information about the binding profile of specific drugs to these receptors can be obtained with studies of cloned receptors transfected to Chinese hampster ovarian (CHO) cells. The binding profile of various representative compounds at the D_2, D_3, and D_4 receptor is illustrated in Table 4–1. Clozapine, the prototypical atypical neuroleptic, has a higher relative affinity for the D_4 receptor compared with the D_2 by a factor of 2.8. Chlorpromazine, which is also an effective antipsychotic agent but with a moderate level of EPS and dyskinesias, presents the inverse profile. Based on the profile of these compounds and the differential localization of the DA-receptor subtypes, R. A. Lahti and colleagues (1993) speculated that dominant D_4-receptor selectivity may confer antipsychotic activity, whereas DA D_2 affinity may confer side-effect activity. To extend these findings, the affinities of a number of antagonists for the D_2 and D_4 receptors were determined using cloned receptors. Plotting the –log ratio of D_2 versus D_4 resulted in the graph shown in Figure 4–3, which represents compounds that are selective for either the D_4 or the D_2 receptor. Among the D_2 receptor–selective drugs, a relationship exists between threshold clinical dose and association with parkinsonism/akathisia.

Hypothetical Experimental Strategies

Because the pathophysiology of schizophrenia is unknown, drug development can only proceed along the line of those strategies that have been successful or new strategies based on speculative ideas of disease pathophysiology. Hypotheses of schizophrenia have involved neurochemical imbalance such as DA overactivity (Carlsson and Lindqvist 1963) or glutamate hypofunction (Kim et al. 1980). Other hypotheses have focused on brain regional

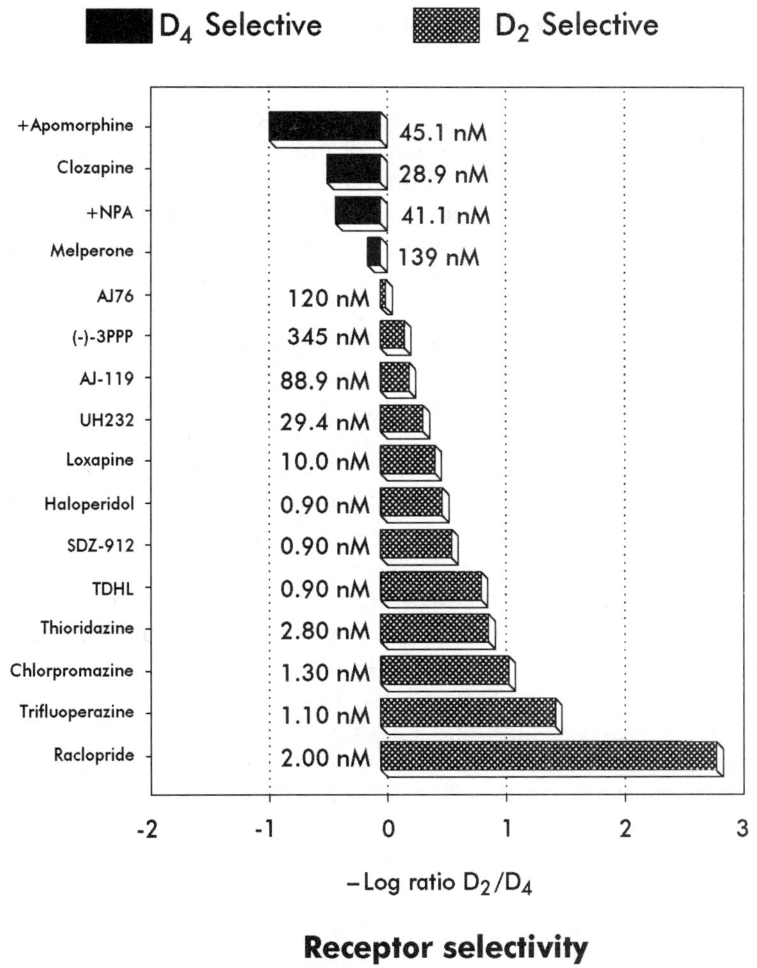

Figure 4–3. Dopamine D_4- and D_2-receptor selectivity for various dopaminergic agents in cloned receptor membrane preparations. NPA = N-propylnorapomorphine.

pathology such as the limbic system (Benes and Bird 1987; Stevens 1973; Tamminga et al. 1992c), frontal cortical function (Selemon et al. 1993; Weinberger et al. 1986), or the basal ganglia (Buchsbaum et al. 1992; Early et al. 1987).

Glutamatergic Treatment

More than 25 years ago, it was observed that phencyclidine (PCP) could mimic the signs and symptoms of schizophrenia (Luby et al. 1959; Pearlson 1981). At psychotomimetic doses, PCP is thought to act selectively at the ion-channel site of the *N*-methyl-D-aspartate (NMDA)-sensitive glutamate receptor, producing blockade of NMDA-sensitive glutamatergic transmission. Various data suggest that glutamatergic transmission may be involved in schizophrenia. Kim et al. (1980) reported a reduced glutamate level in the CSF of patients with schizophrenia. These results, however, have not been consistently replicated (Gattaz et al. 1985; Korpi et al. 1987; Macciardi et al. 1990). Change in the density of different glutamate receptors in different regions of the brain has rather consistently been reported in postmortem studies of patients with schizophrenia (Deakin et al. 1989; Kerwin and Beats 1990; Kornhuber et al. 1989; Kurumaji et al. 1992; Nishikawa et al. 1983; Suga et al. 1990; Toru et al. 1988; Ulas and Cotman 1993).

In 1959, Luby and colleagues gave PCP to patients with schizophrenia and described an overall worsening of their symptoms. To test the hypothesis that PCP may worsen the symptoms of schizophrenia more specifically than other psychotomimetic agents, we gave ketamine, an agonist at the PCP receptor and a structural analogue of PCP, to patients with schizophrenia. Nine patients with schizophrenia voluntarily agreed to participate in this protocol. They were informed about the risks, including the possibility of symptoms worsening. All were taking haloperidol (0.3 mg/kg) at the time of the protocol. Each received, in a double-blind design, three subanesthetic doses of ketamine (0.1, 0.3, and 0.5 mg/kg) and a placebo. Patients had a dose-related, short-lasting (10- to 30-minute) increase in psychotic symptoms. Furthermore, there was a striking similarity between symptoms triggered by ketamine and the delusions the patients presented in the past and/or that were reactivated during medication withdrawal (A. C. Lahti et al. 1995). Overall, studies in this area tend to implicate a reduction in cortical glutamatergic transmission in the pathophysiology of schizophrenia. If so, pharmacological manipulation at the NMDA receptor might be therapeutic. Because of the neurodegenerative potential of direct NMDA receptor stimulation (Schwarcz 1993), indirect functional enhancement of

NMDA-associated transmission may be the most effective pharmacological approach.

The NMDA-PCP receptor is pharmacologically complex and therefore rich for drug targeting. The NMDA receptor regulates ion flow through a Ca^{2+}/K^{+} channel that is voltage regulated and gated by the NMDA receptor. Several additional receptor sites and ions modulate NMDA- and PCP-mediated neurotransmission (Javitt and Zukin 1991). Glycine or its agonist, as well as polyamines, enhance the action of glutamate at the NMDA receptor. Zn^{2+} and Mg^{2+} inhibit flow through the channel; kynurenic acid antagonizes the binding of ligands to the NMDA and glycine sites. Thus, various strategies can affect glutamatergic transmission. For example, glycine agonists or the polyamine spermidine, through potentiation of the action of endogenous NMDA ligands, is an indirect-acting PCP antagonist.

Milacemide is a glycine prodrug; it is metabolized into glycine once it crosses the blood-brain barrier into the CNS. Thus, it presumably might augment the action of glycine at the NMDA-PCP receptor complex. In a crossover, placebo-controlled, double-blind study, milacemide was given to a few patients with schizophrenia who had been withdrawn from their medication for at least 4 weeks. The order of the drug and placebo was random. The effects of milacemide on mental status in the first three subjects who completed this protocol suggested no antipsychotic action (Tamminga et al. 1992a).

Glycine itself, at very high doses, was given as an add-on medication to patients with schizophrenia. Potkin et al. (1992) reported an increased antipsychotic effect with glycine. In a second study, glycine reduced negative symptoms but not positive symptoms of schizophrenia (Zukin 1993). Further studies examining the effect of glycine alone must be carried out to confirm these studies.

Sigma Binding Site Therapeutics

Other psychotomimetic drugs exert their psychosis effect purportedly at the sigma binding site, and those effects are blocked with a sigma antagonist. The sigma "receptor" may be only a poorly defined binding site; its behavioral significance is as yet unknown. Some researchers speculated that a blockade of endogenous sigma ligand may be a treatment for psychosis. Although several traditional neuroleptics have sigma ligand affinity, not all have significant sigma antagonism, and none are relatively selective. BMY 14802 has receptor affinity for the sigma receptor, with some degree of 5-HT_{1a}- and negligible DA-receptor affinity. It did not improve acute exacerbations of symptoms in patients with schizophrenia in an uncontrolled, 4-week study (Gewirtz et al. 1994). NE100, a compound undergoing development, has relatively selective sigma antagonistic influence.

Summary

Antipsychotic drug development has always been and remains challenging. Because the pathophysiology of schizophrenia is unknown, therapeutic agents cannot be directly developed. Animal models do not exist for schizophrenia either, because hallmarks of the illness necessarily involve language. The fact that it is such a pressing medical problem accounts for the vigor of research in this area, despite the hardship.

Current research has produced new compounds for actual and potential use in the treatment of schizophrenia. The characteristics of these drugs are based on aspects of the traditional neuroleptics as well as new dimensions. Opportunity exists to identify unique and improved antipsychotic strategies. The rate of drug discovery today has increased enormously from a decade ago (Table 4–3), which promises new therapeutic agents for tomorrow. This increased rate of discovery is partially a result of the effort and attention of academia and pharmaceutical companies and also the rapid growth of important neuroscience areas.

Several of the newer strategies have produced test compounds that are ready to be evaluated (Table 4–2). These drugs may be studied for simple antipsychotic action or for special effects in a subject population (e.g., neuroleptic nonresponders or dyskinetic subjects). In addition to compounds currently available, a number of strategies are theoretically derived, with compounds in the "pipeline." Although these drugs may require more time for assessment, the strategies are important. This is a critical time for antipsychotic drug research, and considerable promise for new treatments and new information is in the near future.

Table 4–3. New antipsychotic drugs

Drug	**Action**
Clozapine (Sandoz)	Broad-spectrum antagonist/ atypical activity
Risperidone (Janssen)	D_2/5-HT_2 antagonist
Remoxipride (Astra)	Selective D_2 antagonist
Amisulpride	Selective D_2 antagonist
Amperozide (Kabi Lundbeck)	Weak DA antagonist— 5-HT_2 + D_1 antagonist
Sertindole (Abbott)	Broad-spectrum antagonist/ atypical activity
Seroquel (ICI)	Broad-spectrum antagonist/ atypical activity
Olanzapine (Lilly)	Broad-spectrum antagonist/ atypical activity
BRL 46470 (SmithKline Beecham)	5-HT_3 antagonist
RWJ 37796 (R. W. Johnson)	D_2/5-HT_2 antagonist
MDL 100 907 (Marion Merrell Dow)	5-HT_2 antagonist
FCE 23884/005 (Farmitalia)	D_1 agonist/D_2 antagonist
UH232/AJ76 (Upjohn)	D_3 selective antagonist
SCH 39166 (Schering)	D_1 antagonist
NO 22-0010 (Novo)	D_1 antagonist
(-)-3PPP (Carlsson)	Partial DA agonist
SND 919 (Boehringer/Upjohn)	Partial DA agonist
PD 143188 (Parke-Davis)	Partial DA agonist
SDZ-HDC 912	Partial DA agonist
OPC-4392	Partial DA agonist
B-HT 920	Partial DA agonist
EMD 49980	Partial DA agonist

Note. DA = dopamine.

References

Bannon MJ, Elliott PJ, Alpert JE, et al: Role of endogenous substance P in stress-induced activation of mesocortical dopamine neurons. Nature 306:791–792, 1983

Beinfeld MD, Meyer DK, Eskay RL, et al: The distribution of cholecystokinin immunoreactivity in the central nervous system of the rat as determined by radioimmunoassay. Brain Res 212:51–57, 1981

Benes FM: Myelination of cortical-hippocampal relays during late adolescence. Schizophr Bull 15:585–593, 1989

Benes FM, Bird ED: An analysis of the arrangement of neurons in the cingulate cortex of schizophrenic patients. Arch Gen Psychiatry 44:608–616, 1987

Bergstrom DA, Carlson JH, Bromley SD, et al: Differential electrophysiological effects of -3PPP and its enantiomers on dopamine autoreceptors and postsynaptic receptors. Eur J Pharmacol 13:124:75-84, 1986

Bersani G, Grispini A, Marini S, et al: Neuroleptic-induced extra-pyramidal side effects: clinical perspectives with ritanserin (R 55 667), a new selective 5-HT2 receptor blocking agent. Current Therapeutic Research 40:492–499, 1986

Biederman J, Lerner Y, Belmaker RH, et al: Combination of lithium carbonate and haloperidol in schizo-affective disorder: a controlled study. Arch Gen Psychiatry 36:327–333, 1979

Bird ED, Spokes EGS, Iversen LL: Brain norepinephrine and dopamine in schizophrenia. Science 204:93–94, 1979

Bischoff S: Towards the understanding of the neuroanatomical substrate of schizophrenia: the contribution of savoxepine, in Novel Antipsychotic Drugs. Edited by Meltzer HY. New York, Raven, 1992, pp 117–134

Bogerts B, Meertz E, Schonfeldt-Bausch R: Basal ganglia and schizophrenia. Arch Gen Psychiatry 42:784–791, 1985

Bogerts B, Ashtari M, Degreef G, et al: Reduced temporal limbic structure volumes on magnetic resonance images in first episode schizophrenia. Psychiatry Res 35:1–13, 1990

Borison RL, Pathiraja AP, Diamond BI, et al: Risperidone: clinical safety and efficacy in schizophrenia. Psychopharmacol Bull 28:213–218, 1992

Borison RL, Haverstock S, Pathiraja A, et al: Savoxepine as an atypical neuroleptic (abstract). Schizophr Res 9:233, 1993

Brambilla F, Scarone S, Pugnetti L, et al: Bromocriptine therapy in chronic schizophrenia: effects on symptomology, sleep patterns, and prolactin response to stimulation. Psychiatry Res 8:159–169, 1983

Breier A, Buchanan RW, Elkashef A, et al: Brain morphology and schizophrenia: a magnetic resonance imaging study of limbic, prefrontal cortex, and caudate structures. Arch Gen Psychiatry 49:921–926, 1992

Buchsbaum MS, Haier RJ, Potkin SG, et al: Frontostriatal disorder of cerebral metabolism in never-medicated schizophrenics. Arch Gen Psychiatry 49:935–942, 1992

Bunney BS: Antipsychotic drug effects on the electrical activity of dopaminergic neurons. Trends Neurosci 7:212–215, 1984

Carlsson A, Lindqvist M: Effect of chlorpromazine or haloperidol on formation of 3methoxytyramine and normetanephrine in mouse brain. Acta Pharmacologica et Toxicologica 20:140–144, 1963

Carlsson M, Svensson A, Carlsson A: Synergistic interactions between muscarinic antagonists, adrenergic agonists and NMDA antagonists with respect to locomotor stimulatory effects in monoamine-depleted mice. Naunyn Schmiedebergs Arch Pharmacol 343:568–573, 1991

Caron MG, Lefkowitz RJ: Catecholamine receptors: structure, function, and regulation. Recent Prog Horm Res 48:277–290, 1993

Cascella NG, Tarazi FI, Shirakawa O, et al: Savoxepine fails to selectively influence glucose metabolism in the rat limbic system. Psychopharmacology (Berl) 114:275–280, 1994

Chouinard G, Jones B, Remington G, et al: A Canadian multicenter placebo-controlled study of fixed doses of risperidone and haloperidol in the treatment of chronic schizophrenic patients (published erratum). J Clin Psychopharmacol 13:149, 1993

Claghorn JG, Honigfeld G, Abuzzahab FS, et al: The risks and benefits of clozapine versus chlorpromazine. J Clin Psychopharmacol 7:377–384, 1987

Colter N, Battal S, Crow TJ, et al: White matter reduction in the parahippocampal gyrus of patients with schizophrenia (letter). Arch Gen Psychiatry 44:1023, 1987

Conley R, Tamminga CA: Clinical action of remoxipride (letter). Arch Gen Psychiatry 51:1001, 1994

Corsini GU, Del Zompo M, Manconi S, et al: Sedative, hypnotic and antipsychotic effects of low doses of apomorphine in man. Adv Biochem Psychopharmacol 16:645–649, 1977

Corsini GU, Piccardi MP, Bocchetta A, et al: Behavioural effects of apomorphine in men: dopamine receptor implications, in Apomorphine and Other Dopaminomimetics, Vol 2: Clinical Pharmacology. Edited by Corsini GU, Gessa GL. New York, Raven, 1981, pp 13–24

Coward DM: General pharmacology of clozapine. Br J Psychiatry 160:5–11, 1992

Crane GE: Iproniazid phosphate, a therapeutic agent for mental disorders and debilitating disease. Psychiatry Res 8:142–152, 1959

Crawley JN, Vanderhaegen JJ: Potentiation of dopamine-mediated behaviors by CCK in the nucleus accumbens, in Neuronal Cholecystokinin. Edited by Crawlet JN, Vanderhaegen JJ. Ann N Y Acad Sci 448:1–8, 1985

Creese I, Burt DR, Snyder SH: Dopamine receptor binding predicts clinical and pharmacological potencies of antischizophrenic drugs. Science 192:481–483, 1976

Crow TJ, Baker HF, Cross AJ, et al: Monoamine mechanisms in chronic schizophrenia: postmortem neurochemical findings. Br J Psychiatry 134:249–256, 1979

Csernansky JG, Riney SJ, Lombrozo L, et al: Double-blind comparison of alprazolam, diazepam, and placebo for the treatment of negative schizophrenic symptoms. Arch Gen Psychiatry 45:655–659, 1988

Deakin JFW, Slater P, Simpson MDC, et al: Frontal cortical and left temporal glutamatergic dysfunction in schizophrenia. J Neurochem 52:1781–1786, 1989

Delay J, Deniker P: Trente-huit cas de psychoses traitees par la cure prolongee et continue de 4500 R.P. [Thirty-eight cases of psychosis treated by chronic treatment with 4500 R.P.], in Congres des Medecins Alienistes et Neurologistes de France. Edited by Masson P. Luxembourg, 1952, pp 497–502

Deutch AY, Moghaddam B, Innis R, et al: Mechanisms of action of atypical antipsychotic drugs: implications for novel therapeutic strategies for schizophrenia. Schizophr Res 4:121–156, 1991

Douyon R, Angrist B, Peselow E, et al: Neuroleptic augmentation with alprazolam: clinical effects and pharmacokinetic correlates. Am J Psychiatry 146:231–234, 1989

Early TS, Reiman EM, Raichle ME, et al: Left globus pallidus abnormality in never-medicated patients with schizophrenia. Proc Natl Acad Sci U S A 84:561–563, 1987

Fabre LF Jr: A multicenter, open pilot trial of ICI 204,636 in hospitalized patients with acute psychotic symptomology (abstract). Schizophr Res 9:237, 1993

Falkai P, Bogerts B: Cell loss in the hippocampus of schizophrenics. Eur Arch Psychiatry Clin Neurosci 236:154–161, 1986

Farde L, von Bahr C: Distribution of remoxipride to the human brain and central D_2-dopamine receptor binding examined in vivo by PET. Acta Psychiatr Scand 82 (suppl 358):67–71, 1990

Farley IJ, Price KS, McCullough E: Norepinephrine in chronic paranoid schizophrenia: above-normal levels in limbic forebrain. Science 200:456–458, 1978

Ferrier EC, Johnstone EC, Crow TJ: Hormonal effects of apomorphine in schizophrenia. Br J Psychiatry 144:341–348, 1984

Filip V, Marsalek M, Halkova E, et al: Treatment of extrapyramidal side effects with Terguride. Psychiatry Res 41:9–16, 1992

Frey P, Lis M, Coward DM: Neurotensin concentrations in rat striatum and nucleus accumbens: further studies of their regulation. Neurochem Int 12:33–38, 1988

Garver DL, Bissette G, Yao JK, et al: Relation of CSF neurotensin concentrations to symptoms and drug response in psychotic patients. Am J Psychiatry 148:484–488, 1991

Gattaz WF, Riederer P, Reynolds GP, et al: Dopamine and noradrenaline in the cerebrospinal fluid of schizophrenic patients. Psychiatry Res 8:243–250, 1983

Gattaz WF, Gasser T, Beckmann H: Multidimensional analysis of the concentrations of 17 substances in the CSF of schizophrenics and controls. Biol Psychiatry 20:360–366, 1985

Gelders Y, VandenBussche G, Reyntijens A, et al: Serotonin-S2 receptor blockers in the treatment of chronic schizophrenia. Clin Neuropharmacol 9:325–327, 1986

Gerbaldo H, Demisch L, Lehmann CO, et al: The effect of OPC-4392, a partial dopamine receptor agonist on negative symptoms: results of an open study. Pharmacopsychiatry 21:387–388, 1988

Gewirtz GR, Gorman JM, Volavko J, et al: BMY 14802 a sigma receptor ligand for the treatment of schizophrenia. Neuropsychopharmacology 10:37–40, 1994

Gomes UCR, Shanley BC, Potgieter L, et al: Noradrenergic overactivity in chronic schizophrenia: evidence based on cerebrospinal fluid noradrenergic and cyclic nucleotide concentrations. Br J Psychiatry 137: 346–351, 1980

Govoni S, Hong JS, Yang H-YT, et al: Increase of neurotensin content elicited by neuroleptics in nucleus accumbens. J Pharmacol Exp Ther 215:413–417, 1980

Harrison DA, Saherlee W, Tron P, et al: Olanzapine: a potential "atypical" antipsychotic agent—phase II clinical findings (abstract). Schizophr Res 11:107, 1994

Herve D, Simon H, Blanc G, et al: Opposite changes in dopamine utilization in the nucleus accumbens and the frontal cortex after electrolytic lesion of the median raphe in the rat. Brain Res 216:422–428, 1981

Hirschowitz J, Casper R, Garver DL, et al: Lithium response in good prognosis schizophrenia. Am J Psychiatry 137:916–920, 1980

Hokfelt T, Rehfeld L, Skirboll B, et al: Evidence for coexistence of dopamine and CCK in meso-limbic neurons. Nature 285:476–478, 1980

Hommer DW, Pickar D, Roy A, et al: The effects of ceruletide in schizophrenia. Arch Gen Psychiatry 41:617–622, 1984

Janssen PA, Niemegeers CJ, Awouters F, et al: Pharmacology of risperidone (R 64 766), a new antipsychotic with serotonin-S2 and dopamine-D2 antagonistic properties. J Pharmacol Exp Ther 244:685–693, 1988

Javitt DC, Zukin SR: Recent advances in the phencyclidine model of schizophrenia. Am J Psychiatry 148:1301–1308, 1991

Jeste DV, Lohr JB: Hippocampal pathologic findings in schizophrenia. Arch Gen Psychiatry 46:1019–1026, 1989

Jeste DV, Zalcman S, Weinberger DR, et al: Apomorphine response and subtyping of schizophrenia. Prog Neuropsychopharmacol Biol Psychiatry 7:83–88, 1983

Kane J, Honigfeld G, Singer J, et al: Clozapine for the treatment-resistant schizophrenic: a double-blind comparison with chlorpromazine. Arch Gen Psychiatry 45:789–796, 1988

Kebabian JW, Calne DB: Multiple receptors for dopamine. Nature 277:93–96, 1979

Kemali D, Del Vecchio M, Maj M: Increased noradrenaline levels in CSF and plasma of schizophrenic patients. Biol Psychiatry 17:711–717, 1982

Kenakin TP: Efficacy, in Pharmacologic Analysis of Drug Receptor Interaction. New York, Raven, 1993, pp 249–277

Kennedy JL, Petronis A, Macciardi F, et al: The dopamine D_4 receptor and schizophrenia (abstract). Schizophr Res 11:145, 1994

Kerwin RW, Beats BC: Increased forskolin binding in the left parahippocampal gyrus and CA_1 region in postmortem brain determined by quantitative autoradiography. Neurosci Lett 118:164–168, 1990

Kerwin RW, Patel S, Meldrum BS, et al: Asymmetrical loss of glutamate receptor subtype in left hippocampus in schizophrenia. Lancet i:583–584, 1988

Kerwin R, Patel S, Meldrum B: Quantitative autoradiographic analysis of glutamate binding sites in the hippocampal formation in normal and schizophrenic brain postmortem. Neuroscience 39:25–32, 1990

Kilts CD, Anderson CM, Bissette G, et al: Differential effects of antipsychotic drugs on the neurotensin content of discrete brain nuclei. Biochem Pharmacol 37:1547–1554, 1988

Kim JS, Kornhuber HH, Schmid-Beugk W, et al: Low cerebrospinal fluid glutamate in schizophrenic patients and a new hypothesis on schizophrenia. Neurosci Lett 20:379–382, 1980

Kleinman JE, Bridge P, Karoum F, et al: Catecholamines and metabolites in the brains of psychotics and normals: postmortem studies, in Catecholamines: Basic and Clinical Frontiers, Vol 1. Edited by Usdin E, Kopin IJ, Barchas J. Elmsford, NY, Pergamon, 1979, pp 1845–1847

Kline NS: Clinical experience with isoniazid. Journal of Clinical Experimental Psychopathology 19:72–78, 1958

Kohler C, Hall H, Mangnusson O, et al: Biochemical pharmacology of the atypical neuroleptic remoxipride. Acta Psychiatr Scand Suppl 102:27–36, 1990

Kornhuber J, Mack-Burkhardt F, Riederer P, et al: [^{3}H] MK-801 binding sites in postmortem brain regions of schizophrenic patients. J Neural Transm Gen Sect 77:231–236, 1989

Korpi ER, Kaufmann CA, Marnela KM, et al: Cerebrospinal fluid amino acid concentrations in chronic schizophrenia. Psychiatr Res 20:337–345, 1987

Kovelman JA, Scheibel AB: A neurohistological correlate of schizophrenia. Biol Psychiatry 19:1601–1619, 1984

Kurumaji A, Ishimaru M, Toru M: α-[^{3}H]Amino-3-hydroxy-5-methylisoxazole-4-propionic acid binding to human cerebral cortical membranes: minimal changes in postmortem brains of chronic schizophrenics. J Neurochem 59:829–837, 1992

Lader MH: Neuroleptic-induced deficit syndrome (NIDS). J Clin Psychiatry 54:493–500, 1993

Lahti AC, Koffel BL, LaPorte D, et al: Subanesthetic doses of ketamine stimulate psychosis in schizophrenia. Neuropsychopharmacology 13:9–19, 1995

Lahti RA, Evans DL, Stratman NC, et al: Dopamine D_4 versus D_2 receptor selectivity of dopamine receptor antagonists: possible therapeutic implications. Eur J Pharmacol 236:483–486, 1993

Lake CR, Sternberg D, van Kammen DP, et al: Schizophrenia: elevated cerebrospinal fluid norepinephrine. Science 207:331–333, 1980

Levy MI, Davis BM, Mohs RC, et al: Apomorphine and schizophrenia. Arch Gen Psychiatry 41:520–524, 1984

Lewander T, Westerbergh SE, Morrison D: Clinical profile of remoxipride: a combined analysis of a comparative double-blind multicentre trial programme. Acta Psychiatr Scand Suppl 358:92–98, 1990

Leysen JC, Gommeren W, Eens A, et al: Biochemical profile of risperidone, a new antipsychotic. J Pharmacol Exp Ther 247:661–670, 1988

Lindstrom LH, Widerlov E, Bissette G, et al: Reduced CSF neurotensin concentration in drug-free schizophrenic patients. Schizophr Res 1:55–59, 1988

Litman RE, Hong WW, Weissman EM, et al: Idazoxan, an α_2 antagonist, augments fluphenazine response in schizophrenic patients: a pilot study. J Clin Psychopharmacol 13:264–267, 1993

Lotstra F, Verbanck P, Mendelewicz J, et al: No evidence of antipsychotic effect of caerulein in schizophrenic patients free of neuroleptics: a double-blind crossover study. Biol Psychiatry 6:877–882, 1984

Luby ED, Cohen BD, Rosenbaum G, et al: Study of a new schizophrenomimetic drug—sernyl. Arch Gen Psychiatry 81:363–369, 1959

Macciardi F, Lucca A, Catalano M, et al: Amino acid patterns in schizophrenia: some new findings. Psychiatry Res 32:63–70, 1990

Marder SR: Risperidone: clinical development: North American results. Clin Neuropharmacol 15 (suppl 1 pt A):92A–93A, 1992

Martin PT, Grebb JA, Schmitz PJ, et al: Efficacy and safety of sertindole in double-blind, placebo-controlled trials of schizophrenic patients (abstract). Schizophr Res 11:107, 1994

McLean S, Ganong AH, Seeger TF, et al: Activity and distribution of binding sites in brain of a nonpeptide substance P (NK1) receptor antagonist. Science 251:437–439, 1991

Meltzer HY: Relevance of dopamine autoreceptors for psychiatry: preclinical and clinical studies. Schizophr Bull 6:456–475, 1980

Meltzer HY: Clinical studies on the mechanism of action of clozapine: the dopamine-serotonin hypothesis of schizophrenia. Psychopharmacology (Berl) 99:S18–S27, 1989

Meltzer HY, Burnett S, Bastani B, et al: Effects of six months of clozapine treatment on the quality of life of chronic schizophrenic patients. Hosp Community Psychiatry 41:892–897, 1990

Moore NA, Tye NC, Axton MS, et al: The behavioral pharmacology of olanzapine, a novel "atypical" antipsychotic agent. J Pharmacol Exp Ther 262:545–551, 1992

Naber D: Efficacy and tolerability of the partial dopamine agonist SDZ-HDC-912 in the treatment of schizophrenia (abstract). Schizophr Res 4:323, 1991

Nemeroff CB, Youngblood W, Manberg PJ, et al: Regional brain concentrations of neuropeptides in Huntington's chorea and schizophrenia. Science 221:972–975, 1983

Nicolaou NM, Garcia-Munoz M, Arbuthnott GW, et al: Interactions between serotonergic and dopaminergic systems in rat brain demonstrated by small unilateral lesions of the raphe nuclei. Eur J Pharmacol 57:295–305, 1979

Nishikawa T, Takashima M, Toru M: Increased [^{3}H]-kainic acid binding in the prefrontal cortex in schizophrenia. Neurosci Lett 40:245–250, 1983

Ohmori T, Koyama T, Inoue T, et al: B-HT 920, a dopamine D_2 agonist in the treatment of negative symptoms of chronic schizophrenia. Biol Psychiatry 33:687–693, 1993

Olbrich R, Schanz H: The effect of the partial dopamine agonist terguride on negative symptoms in schizophrenics. Pharmacopsychiatry 21:389–390, 1988

Pakkenberg B: Pronounced reduction of total neuron number in mediodorsal thalamic nucleus and nucleus accumbens in schizophrenics. Arch Gen Psychiatry 47:1023–1027, 1990

Pearlson GD: Psychiatric and medical syndromes associated with phencyclidine (PCP) abuse. Johns Hopkins Medical Journal 148:25–33, 1981

Peroutka SJ, Snyder SH: Relationship of neuroleptic drug effects at brain dopamine, serotonin, α-adrenergic, and histamine receptors to clinical potency. Am J Psychiatry 137:1518–1522, 1980

Potkin SG, Costa J, Roy S, et al: Glycine in the treatment of schizophrenia: theory and preliminary results, in Novel Antipsychotic Drugs. Edited by Meltzer HY. New York, Raven, 1992, pp 179–188

Potkin SG, Anand R, Sandoz Collaborating Centers: A partial dopamine agonist SDZ HDC 912 has antipsychotic efficacy (abstract). Schizophr Res 9:247, 1993

Prusoff BA, Williams DH, Weissman MM, et al: Treatment of secondary depression in schizophrenia: a double-blind, placebo-controlled trial of amitriptyline added to perphenazine. Arch Gen Psychiatry 36:569–575, 1979

Rasmussen K, Aghajanian GK: Potency of antipsychotics in reversing the effects of a hallucinogenic drug on locus coeruleus neurons correlates with 5-HT_2 binding affinity. Neuropsychopharmacology 1:101–107, 1988

Roberts GW, Ferrier IN, Lee Y, et al: Peptides, the limbic lobe and schizophrenia. Brain Res 288:199–211, 1983

Scheibel AB, Kovelman JA: Disorientation of the hippocampal pyramidal cell and its processes in schizophrenia patients. Biol Psychiatry 16:101–102, 1981

Schwarcz R: Metabolism and function of brain kynurenines. Biochem Soc Trans 21:77–82, 1993

Seeman P, Lee T, Chau-Wong M, et al: Antipsychotic drug doses and neuroleptic/dopamine receptors. Nature 261:717–719, 1976

Seeman P, Guan HC, Van Tol HHM: Dopamine D_4 receptors elevated in schizophrenia. Nature 365:441–446, 1993

Selemon LD, Rajkowska G, Goldman-Rakic PS: A morphometric analysis of prefrontal areas 9 and 40 in the schizophrenic and normal human brain (abstract). Schizophr Res 9:151, 1993

Siris SG, van Kammen DP, Docherty JP: Use of antidepressant drugs in schizophrenia. Arch Gen Psychiatry 35:1368–1377, 1978

Siris SG, Rifkin A, Reardon GT, et al: A trial of adjunctive imipramine in post-psychotic depression. Psychopharmacol Bull 21:114–116, 1985

Skarsfeldt T, Perregaard J: Sertindole, a new neuroleptic with extreme selectivity on A10 versus A9 dopamine neurons in the rat. Eur J Pharmacol 182:613–614, 1990

Small JG, Kellams JJ, Milstein V, et al: A placebo-controlled study of lithium combined with neuroleptics in chronic schizophrenic patients. Am J Psychiatry 132:1315–1317, 1975

Snyder SH, Creese I, Burt D: The brain's dopamine receptor: labeling with [^{3}H]dopamine and [^{3}H]haloperidol. Psychopharmacological Communications 1:663–673, 1975

Stevens JR: An anatomy of schizophrenia? Arch Gen Psychiatry 29:177–189, 1973

Stowe ZN, Nemeroff CB: Nondopaminergic mechanisms relevant to antipsychotic activity, in New Generation of Antipsychotic Drugs: Novel Mechanism of Actions, Vol 4. Edited by Brunello N, Menlewicz J, Racagni G. Basel, Karger, 1993, pp 15–26

Suddath RL, Casanova MF, Goldberg TE, et al: Temporal lobe pathology in schizophrenia: a quantitative magnetic resonance imaging study. Am J Psychiatry 146:464–472, 1989

Suga I, Kogayashi T, Ogata H, et al: Increased 3H-MK801 binding in postmortem brains of chronic schizophrenic patients (abstract). The Satellite Symposium of the 17th Collegium Internationale Neuropsychopharmacologicum, 1990, p 28

Svensson K, Carlsson A: Animal data in support of the treatment of EPS with partial dopamine receptor agonists (abstract). Schizophr Res 9:253, 1993

Svensson L, Ahlenius S: Suppression of exploratory locomotor activity in the rat by the local application of (-)-3PPP into the nucleus accumbens. Eur J Pharmacol 88:393–397, 1983

Tamminga CA, Schaffer MH: Treatment of schizophrenia with ergot derivatives. Psychopharmacology 66:239–242, 1979

Tamminga CA, Schaffer MH, Smith RC, et al: Schizophrenic symptoms improve with apomorphine. Science 200:567–568, 1978

Tamminga CA, Gotts MD, Thaker GK, et al: Dopamine agonist treatment of schizophrenia with N-propylnorapomorphine. Arch Gen Psychiatry 43:398–402, 1986a

Tamminga CA, Littman RL, Alphs LD, et al: Cholecystokinin: a neuropeptide in the treatment of schizophrenia. Psychopharmacology (Berl) 88:387–391, 1986b

Tamminga CA, Cascella N, Fakouhi TD, et al: Enhancement of NMDA-mediated transmission in schizophrenia, in Novel Antipsychotic Drugs. Edited by Meltzer HY. New York, Raven, 1992a, pp 171–177

Tamminga CA, Cascella NG, Lahti RA, et al: Pharmacologic properties of (-)-3PPP (preclamol) in man. J Neural Transm Gen Sect 88:165–175, 1992b

Tamminga CA, Thaker GK, Buchanan R, et al: Limbic system abnormalities identified in schizophrenia using positron emission tomography with fluorodeoxyglucose and neocortical alterations with deficit syndrome. Arch Gen Psychiatry 49:522–530, 1992c

Tanaka K, Masu M, Nakarishi S: Structure and functional expression of the cloned rat neurotensin receptor. Neuron 4:847–854, 1990

Toru M, Watanabe S, Shibuya H, et al: Neurotransmitters, receptors and neuropeptides in post-mortem brains of chronic schizophrenic patients. Acta Psychiatr Scand 78:121–137, 1988

Ulas J, Cotman CW: Excitatory amino acid receptors in schizophrenia. Schizophr Bull 19:105–117, 1993

Van Tol HHM, Bunzow JR, Guan HC, et al: Cloning of the gene for a human dopamine D_4 receptor with high affinity for the antipsychotic clozapine. Nature 350:610, 1991

Van Tol HHM, Wu CM, Guan HC, et al: Multiple dopamine D_4 receptor variants in the human population. Nature 358:149–152, 1992

Waehrens J, Gerlach J: Antidepressant drugs in anergic schizophrenia: a double-blind cross over study with maprotiline and placebo. Acta Psychiatr Scand 61:438–444, 1980

Weinberger DR, Berman KF, Zee RF: Physiologic dysfunction of dorsolateral prefrontal cortex in schizophrenia, I: regional cerebral blood flow evidence. Arch Gen Psychiatry 43:114–124, 1986

Wetzel H, Benkert O: Dopamine autoreceptor agonists in the treatment of schizophrenic disorders. Prog Neuropsychopharmacol Biol Psychiatry 17:525–540, 1993

Widerlov E, Lindstrom LH, Besev G, et al: Subnormal CSF levels of neurotensin in a subgroup of schizophrenic patients: normalization after neuroleptic treatment. Am J Psychiatry 139:1122–1126, 1982

Wiedemann K, Benkert O, Holsboer F: B-HT 920—a novel dopamine autoreceptor agonist in the treatment of patients with schizophrenia. Pharmacopsychiatry 23:50–55, 1990

Wiedemann K, Krieg JC, Loyche A, et al: Novel dopamine autoreceptor agonists B-HT 920 and EMD 49980 in the treatment of patients with schizophrenia, in Novel Antipsychotic Drugs. Edited by Meltzer HY. New York, Raven, 1992, pp 91–98

Wolkowitz OM, Breier A, Doran A, et al: Alprazolam augmentation of the antipsychotic effects of fluphenazine in schizophrenic patients: preliminary results. Arch Gen Psychiatry 45:664–671, 1988

Zukin S: The effects of glycine on negative symptoms of schizophrenia. Presented at the University of Maryland, Department of Psychiatry Ground Rounds, Baltimore, MD, November 1993

CHAPTER 5

Conventional Neuroleptic Treatment: Current Status, Future Role

John M. Kane, M.D.

Clinicians' understanding of schizophrenia has greatly improved; however, the treatment of this disease continues to challenge mental health professionals. Schizophrenia is a complex disease that manifests in cognitive, behavioral, and psychosocial symptoms. It requires health care professionals to integrate and address biological, psychosocial, and environmental influences. Despite the numerous advances in various research areas ranging from brain imaging and genetics to neurochemistry and neuropharmacology, the psychopharmacological agents routinely used to treat schizophrenia have not changed dramatically over the past 30 years. Significant progress has been made in our ability to diagnose conditions in patients using established, valid, and reliable criteria. Significantly greater numbers of patients with schizophrenia are maintained in the community, with varying degrees of success. Those individuals who do remain in hospitals are likely to be either refractory, violent, or aggressive or to have severe psychosocial and environmental deprivation and lack of support.

In recent years, clinical psychopharmacological research has focused on two lines of investigation: 1) to develop better pharmacological agents that might have a broader spectrum of activity and/or a superior benefit-to-risk ratio and 2) to improve our ability to use available pharmacotherapeutic agents in the most effective and least toxic fashion. As discussed elsewhere in this volume, the recent introduction of clozapine and the development of other potential atypical antipsychotic drugs has stimulated renewed interest in drug development and has provided increased optimism as to the potential for developing better compounds.

In this chapter, I discuss the current status of conventional neuroleptic treatment, highlight recent developments and prospects for future advancement, and identify areas that need further clinical investigation.

Acute Treatment

The acute treatment phase in the pharmacotherapy of schizophrenia suggests the introduction or reintroduction of medication to treat a relapse or exacerbation in psychosis. As a rule, these episodes result from a discontinuation of medication or the impact of a stressful life event, although some relapses occur for reasons that are not obvious to the treating clinician. These episodes are usually indicated by an increase in positive symptoms such as delusions, hallucinations, thought disorder or agitation, and aggressive behavior. However, in some patients an increase in negative symptoms such as extreme withdrawal and uncommunicativeness might also occur.

Episodes vary enormously in their rapidity of onset as well as in the form and content of the symptoms. The presentation may change over time and may be influenced by a variety of factors.

The role of antipsychotic drug treatment in the management of an acute episode of schizophrenia has been well established over the past several decades. Conventional neuroleptic drugs remain the primary modality in the treatment of an acute episode or an acute exacerbation of a schizophrenic illness.

Unfortunately, despite the proven efficacy of antipsychotic drugs in this context, there is an enormous degree of heterogeneity in drug response, and a substantial proportion of patients derive relatively little, if any, benefit from drug treatment (Davis and Casper 1977). Even among those individuals who do benefit, a large subgroup are left with significant residual symptomatology (both positive and negative). This symptomatology, particularly the negative symptoms, contributes greatly to the persistent disability, subjective distress, and family burden associated with chronic schizophrenia.

Once an appropriate diagnostic evaluation is made, the critical considerations in determining acute pharmacological treatment strategies involve choice of drug, drug dosage, and dosage escalation schedule and potential role of concomitant or adjunctive treatments.

Drug Type

A common assumption is that all antipsychotic agents are equally efficacious. However, data on clozapine (Kane et al. 1988) call this assumption into question. It may be that this assumption has not been tested adequately even with conventional neuroleptic drugs. In general, drugs are compared in large-scale clinical trials, and a percentage of patients responding to one drug is compared with the percentage of patients responding to a second drug. If this ratio is not significantly different, it is assumed that the drugs are equally efficacious. This does not mean, however, that either drug would work equally as well in any individual. Few studies have explored the response to a second drug in patients who have not responded to a first drug (this issue will be discussed further in the context of the treatment of refractory patients).

Most clinicians choose a drug based on several factors. One critical factor should be a detailed history of prior drug treatment and response. If the clinician can elicit evidence that a patient has responded well to a particular drug in the past, this would be the single most important reason to recommend the use of that drug in the future. At the same time, however, clinicians should be careful in accepting at face value a potentially negative report from a patient regarding a prior drug experience. Some patients will say they are "allergic" to a given medication when in fact they had experienced a drug side effect (e.g., a dystonic reaction). If the patient has not been previously treated (and does not have any relatives previously treated for the same condition), no specific predictors would recommend one class of drug over another. Although some clinicians continue to assume that sedatives are more effective for agitated or hyperactive patients, whereas so-called high-potency drugs are more effective for withdrawn and less-active patients, no consistent data support this assumption. Therefore, clinicians will probably use those drugs with which they are most familiar and most comfortable. It is also likely that in the near future cost will play an increasing role in the determination of drug preference.

It is also important for clinicians to consider long-range treatment planning even when initiating acute treatment in the hospital. If the patient has relapsed because of noncompliance, clinicians should carefully consider the possible use of long-acting injectable neuroleptics. Many clinicians tend to reserve so-called guaranteed medication for noncompliant patients with a repeated history of relapse. Because rates of noncompliance have been found to be very high in this patient population, and good predictors are not available for identifying those patients at risk for noncompliance, it would seem logical to consider using long-acting injectable drugs in the majority of patients before relapse potentially resulting from noncompliance (Glazer and Kane 1992). This consideration is important even during the inpatient phase of treatment because after a patient is discharged, it is often difficult for a new treatment team to introduce a change in medication or route of administration. On the other hand, if the patient is educated about the potential advantages of long-acting injectable drugs before discharge and even provided with an initial test dose, this may facilitate a smooth transition from oral to depot treatment.

Drug Dosage

Although the issue of dosage has received increasing attention in recent years, definitive dose response curves are not available for antipsychotic drugs. Although recent research has guided clinicians in determining dosage, individual titration and clinical judgment continue to be important. In the very early stages of antipsychotic drug development, data suggested that doses of chlorpromazine below 400–600 mg/day were much less likely to be superior to placebo in clinical efficacy than doses above that range. Subsequently, considerable attention was given to determining whether very high doses of antipsychotic drug treatment offered any potential benefit in terms of rapidity of therapeutic onset or ultimate degree of improvement (particularly in poor or partial responders). Studies comparing high doses (e.g., greater than 2,000 mg chlorpromazine equivalents) with standard doses did not show any consistent superiority for high-dose treatment (Kane 1987). Some patients may benefit from higher than usual dosages, but currently we do not have any reliable means to identify such individuals, who clearly appear to be in the minority.

Reardon et al. (1989) reported that the use of high dosages of high-potency neuroleptic drugs increased in the late 1970s and 1980s despite the lack of clinical research data supporting such use. This phenomenon may have been a result of clinicians' need to treat patients rapidly and to provide early discharge from the hospital and/or the increasing acuity and severity of symptoms in those individuals being hospitalized. The fact that high-potency drugs are generally well tolerated also contributed to clinicians' relative comfort with these strategies.

Several studies have contributed further information regarding dosage requirements for acute treatment. Levinson et al. (1990) reported on 53 patients with acute exacerbations of schizophrenia and other nonaffective psychoses. Patients were randomly assigned on a double-blind basis to receive fixed-dose treatment with either 10, 20, or 30 mg/day of oral fluphenazine. Following 24–28 days of treatment, the investigators did not find improvement in the sample as a whole to be related to dosage. However, in patients who showed a 40% or greater reduction in positive symptoms, doses greater than 0.3 mg/kg were associated with the greatest clinical improvement. At the same time, however, these doses also produced a higher incidence of extrapyramidal side effects. The investigators concluded that although the best clinical response was observed with doses of 0.3 mg/kg/day, the increase in adverse effects was such that they would recommend lower daily doses in the range of 0.2–0.3 mg/kg. Also note that the investigators reported that the presence of akathisia during the study (regardless of whether the patient was treated for akathisia) also predicted poor response.

Van Putten et al. (1990) studied 80 newly admitted men with

schizophrenia who were openly assigned by cohort to receive 5, 10, or 20 mg/day of haloperidol for 4 weeks. After 1 week of treatment, the percentage of patients who remained in the study and were characterized as "much improved" was 6% for the 5-mg group, 33% for the 10-mg group, and 47% for the 20-mg group. Although the 20-mg daily dose appeared to be superior in efficacy during the first week or two, this group experienced a subsequent worsening in emotional withdrawal and psychomotor retardation as well as a higher incidence of rated akinesia and akathisia. The investigators also reported a 35% dropout rate among the patients receiving the highest dose compared with only 5% for those in the two lower-dose groups. Van Putten and colleagues concluded that 20 mg/day may be more effective for controlling psychosis in the initial phase of the treatment trial, but a subsequent high incidence of adverse effects may undermine this benefit. Note that this was an open study, and the prophylactic or early use of antiparkinsonian agents (or propranolol) could improve the therapeutic index.

Rifkin et al. (1991) randomly assigned 87 newly admitted patients with schizophrenia to receive 10, 30, or 80 mg/day of oral haloperidol on a double-blind basis for 6 weeks. These investigators found no difference in dropout rate, clinical response, or the occurrence of extrapyramidal side effects among the three treatment groups. Rifkin and co-workers concluded that there was no advantage to treating patients with haloperidol doses higher than 10 mg/day, but they also did not find a significant increase in extrapyramidal side effects among patients treated with higher doses and prophylactic antiparkinsonian medication.

There is reasonable agreement across these studies despite differences in patient population and methodology. Therefore, there appear to be no significant advantages to using doses of haloperidol or fluphenazine greater than 10–20 mg/day for acute treatment.

McEvoy et al. (1991) arrived at a somewhat different conclusion using a novel methodology to determine optimal dose in a much younger and more acutely ill population. McEvoy and associates studied the "neuroleptic threshold" hypothesis, which suggests that the lowest neuroleptic doses at which patients develop slight increases in rigidity are the doses at which patients will attain maximum therapeutic benefit.

Of the 106 patients who participated in this study, 25 had schizoaffective disorder and 32 had no prior exposure to neuroleptic drugs. After patients achieved their neuroleptic threshold dose, they were treated openly for 2 weeks and then randomly assigned on a double-blind basis either to continue at the neuroleptic threshold dose or to have the dosage increased by 2–10 times. The average "high" dose between days 24 and 38 was 11.6 mg/day versus 3.4 mg/day for those continuing at their neuroleptic threshold dose (haloperidol was the medication used). It is interesting that neuroleptic-naive patients crossed the threshold at a significantly lower average dose (2.1 mg/day) than those who had been treated previously with neuroleptic drugs (4.3 mg/day). These investigators found no difference between those remaining on the neuroleptic threshold dose and those randomized to a higher dose. The only therapeutic measures on which the higher dose was considered superior were ratings of hostility and suspiciousness. However, at the same time, higher doses were also associated with more extrapyramidal side effects.

The inclusion of more first-episode and drug-naive patients in the McEvoy et al. (1991) study may account for the apparent disparity with the findings of the studies cited earlier in this chapter. Average doses of haloperidol above 11.6 mg/day might have produced better results in those patients initially categorized as nonresponders.

It would appear that there is a strong consensus that doses of haloperidol or fluphenazine above 15–20 mg/day should not be the first-line treatment in patients who are judged to be capable of responding; that is, those without an established history of neuroleptic refractoriness. It is also apparent that side effects associated with antipsychotic drugs, such as akinesia and akathisia, are significant clinical problems even at dosages in the recommended range, and clinicians must be sensitive to the need to prevent and treat them.

Refractory Patients

It is clear that a significant number of individuals with schizophrenia do not respond adequately to a standard trial of antipsychotic drugs. Data from our group (Kinon et al. 1993) suggest that substantially increasing the dosage or switching to a different class of antipsychotic drug does not necessarily bring about further response, although these are the strategies most widely employed in hospital settings. It is likely that some patients are limited in the degree to which they will benefit from typical antipsychotic drugs. This highlights the need for further research to identify factors contributing to nonresponsiveness as well as to develop alternative treatments that might prove more efficacious.

Kinon et al. (1993) have reported on patients with schizophrenia or schizoaffective or schizophreniform disorders treated openly with fluphenazine 20 mg/day for 4 weeks. Those patients who did not meet a priori response criteria and who consented to participate were randomly assigned on a double-blind basis to receive fluphenazine 80 mg/day or haloperidol 20 mg/day or to continue on fluphenazine 20 mg/day. The double-blind phase lasted an additional 4 weeks. Only 7% of those who had not met response criteria after the first 4 weeks responded after 8 weeks of treatment. In addition, no significant differences were found among the three alternatives. Some refractory patients might benefit from substantial increases in dosage or from switching to a different chemical class of antipsychotic drug, but improved methods to identify such patients are necessary before such treatment could be recommended on a broader scale.

Maintenance Treatment

Antipsychotic medications not only play a role in the acute alleviation of psychotic signs and symptoms, but they are also critical in the long-term maintenance treatment of schizophrenia. Their efficacy in this context has been established in numerous clinical trials over the last three decades (Davis 1975; Kane and Lieberman 1987). In the past decade, maintenance-treatment studies have focused increasingly on attempting to improve the benefit-to-risk ratio of long-term treatment. In addition, these studies have explored a variety of alternative maintenance strategies intended to reduce long-term cumulative neuroleptic exposure.

The risk of tardive dyskinesia has been a major impetus for dosage reduction strategies. Also, the clinical awareness that behaviorally manifested adverse effects such as akathisia and akinesia can be a significant problem has contributed to the rationale for such studies. It is likely that a variety of adverse effects, but particularly extrapyramidal side effects, contribute to the high rates of noncompliance in medication taking among patients with schizophrenia.

Two different types of study designs have been employed in an attempt to establish minimum effective dosage requirements for maintenance treatment. The first design was the comparison of different dosages of medication on a double-blind random-assignment basis, and the second design was the comparison of continuous drug treatment with an "intermittent" or "targeted" maintenance strategy.

In considering the respective results of these studies, it is important to keep in mind that outcome measures such as prodromal signs of relapse and psychotic exacerbation may be defined and applied differently in each study. However, despite the potential differences in terms of setting, patient population, methodology, and so forth, a remarkable degree of consistency exists across many of these reports.

Four studies have been published involving outpatients followed for at least 1 year on different randomly assigned dosages of maintenance medication. Kane et al. (1983, 1985) reported on 163 patients who were randomly assigned to one of three dosage ranges of fluphenazine decanoate on a double-blind basis: 1.25–5.0 mg, 2.5–10.0 mg, or 12.5–50 mg given every other week. At the end of 1 year, the cumulative relapse rates defined by a priori Brief Psychiatric Rating Scale (BPRS; Overall and Gorham 1962) criteria involving change in psychotic items were 56% on the lowest dose, 24% on the intermediate dose, and 14% on the highest dose.

Although there was a significantly higher relapse rate among the patients receiving the lowest dose, relatively few had to be rehospitalized, and, on average, patients had returned to their baseline state within 9 weeks of receiving an increase in dosage. Among patients receiving the lower dosage, there was improvement on some measures of psychosocial adjustment as well as ratings of emotional withdrawal, tension, blunted affect, and psychomotor retardation. Although some of these signs are associated with negative symptoms, it appears that their improvement in this context was most likely due to a reduction in extrapyramidal side effects.

Marder et al. (1984, 1987) reported on 66 male outpatients in a Veterans Administration setting who were randomly assigned to receive 5 mg or 25 mg of fluphenazine decanoate every other week; these patients were followed for 2 years. The investigators defined three levels of outcome: psychotic exacerbation, relapse, and rehospitalization. At the end of 1 year, the exacerbation rates were 35% on 5 mg and 43% on 25 mg, whereas the relapse rates were 22% versus 20%. These differences were nonsignificant. However, after 2 years of follow-up, the two dosages resulted in different rates of exacerbation—69% in the 5-mg group compared with 36% in the 25-mg group. These results emphasize the importance of employing a long-term time frame in assessing the relative benefits of different maintenance-treatment strategies. Note that few studies to date have lasted more than 1 year.

Johnson et al. (1987) observed 59 stable schizophrenic outpatients who had been receiving up to 40 mg of flupentixol decanoate every 2 weeks for at least 1 year. Patients were randomly assigned either to continue taking their original dosage or to receive a 50% reduced dosage; all patients were followed for 1 year. A significantly higher (32%) relapse rate was seen in the dosage-reduction group compared with the control subjects (10%). After the first year of the study, those patients originally assigned to continue taking their regular dose also had their dosage reduced by 50%, and all patients were followed for an additional 2 years. Of the patients given the reduced dosage, 70% relapsed after 3 years, and 56% relapsed after 2 years.

Hogarty et al. (1988) studied 70 stable outpatients who were categorized as living in high expressed emotion (EE) or low EE households. Patients participating in this study were randomly assigned on a double-blind basis to receive a standard dose of fluphenazine decanoate (mean 25 mg every 2 weeks) or a minimal dose that was approximately 20% of the original dose (mean 3.8 mg). After 1 year, the relapse rate for patients taking the higher dosage was 14% in comparison to 22% for the lower dosage. After 2 years, the rates were 24% and 30%, respectively. No significant differences in relapse rates were found between dosages at 1 or 2 years. These investigators also reported that the lower dosage showed an advantage in terms of less emotional withdrawal in psychomotor retardation and better psychosocial and vocational adjustment as reported by Kane et al. (1985).

These studies suggest that dosage can be significantly reduced in many patients, but a substantial proportion will relapse. As the dose was decreased and the length of time that patients were followed increased, the relapse rate increased. In addition, it appears that patients who are less stable initially have a greater likelihood of relapse (Hogarty 1984). Although dosage reduction can reduce adverse effects, the reduction in the risk of tardive dyskinesia does not appear to be either consistent or dramatic. A relatively brief, 1- to 2-year, time frame may not be adequate to examine the full impact of these strategies on the long-term risk of tardive dyskinesia, but this remains to be seen. It would also be valuable to identify those patients who are at particularly high risk for the development of tardive dyskinesia and examine whether such strategies have a more obvious effect on reducing their risk.

Targeted or Intermittent Medication

The objectives of this strategy are somewhat similar to those of the previously discussed continuous, low-dose strategy. Overall, the hope is to reduce the risk of tardive dyskinesia and to lessen extrapyramidal and other side effects, with the goal of improved subjective well-being and improved compliance. This strategy entails careful clinical observation for early signs of relapse (so-called prodromal symptoms) and reinstating medication at the earliest possible time.

Herz and Melville (1980) have shown that some patients have a characteristic prodromal period with specific signs and symptoms that can be identified by clinicians and families as precursors of decompensation.

Four major studies have been reported on targeted or intermittent treatment. Herz et al. (1991) conducted a double-blind study involving 140 patients who had been stable and out of the hospital. They were withdrawn from medication for 8 weeks on a single-blind basis. Twenty percent of the subjects experienced prodromal episodes during this period and were excluded from further study. This is an important point in terms of the generalizability of this approach to an unselected population of outpatients with schizophrenia. One hundred one patients were then randomly assigned to restart medication or to receive placebo. If a patient experienced a prodromal episode, active open medication was reinstituted. Once the patient was stabilized, blinded study treatment was continued and open medication discontinued. Intermittently treated patients did receive significantly less medication; however, they were also significantly less likely to complete the 2-year study (38% versus 72%) in comparison to those receiving continuous treatment. Many patients were dropped from the study because they experienced three or more prodromal episodes in 1 year. Patients receiving continuous medication lasted significantly longer periods of time without either prodromal episodes or full relapses.

Carpenter et al. (1990) published a report involving 116 newly discharged patients. Following a 4- to 8-week stabilization period and a 4-week medication discontinuation period, subjects participating in the study were randomly assigned to receive either continuous treatment or targeted treatment for a 2-year period. The treatment administered was not blind. Targeted treatment patients received medication for only 52% of the time; however, significantly greater numbers of patients in the continuous treatment group completed the entire 2-year trial. Patients who received targeted treatment experienced significantly more clinical decompensations and were more likely to be hospitalized. Among those individuals who remained in treatment after 2 years, the degree of job employment was significantly better among continuously treated patients.

A study conducted in England (Jolley et al. 1989, 1990) involved 54 outpatients with schizophrenia who had been stable for at least 6 months and on injectable fluphenazine decanoate for at least 2 months. Subjects were randomly assigned on a double-blind basis either to continue medication or to have placebo substituted for active drug. The trial was 2 years in duration. Investigators reported no difference in the number of patients completing the first year of the trial; however, significantly more patients receiving the intermittent treatment (76%) experienced prodromal episodes compared with those receiving continuous treatment (27%). The intermittent group also experienced a significantly greater number of relapses, but the number of hospitalizations did not differ between the two groups. In the second year, both rates of relapse and rehospitalization were significantly greater among those in the intermittent group. Although there had been a trend toward a reduced incidence of tardive dyskinesia in the intermittent group at the end of 1 year, this difference was not seen at the end of the second year.

In a German sample (Pietzcker et al. 1986), standard maintenance medication, neuroleptic crisis intervention, and prophylactic early neuroleptic intervention were compared. The investigators studied 365 patients from four different clinical settings. Patients participating were required to have a 3-month period of stabilization after discharge from the hospital. After both 1 and 2 years, those subjects receiving early intervention treatment had significantly higher relapse rates compared with those receiving standard maintenance treatment. The rate of rehospitalization was not significantly greater in the first year (23% versus 16%) but did reach significance in the second year (37% versus 24%). Patients receiving only neuroleptic crisis intervention had a higher relapse rate than the other two groups.

There are some important differences in these studies. For example, the Herz et al. (1991) and Jolley et al. studies were double-blind, whereas the other two studies were not. Despite this, considerable agreement exists in the overall conclusions. It is safe to suggest that intermittent-treatment strategies can be implemented in an outpatient setting and can result in reduced cumulative neuroleptic exposure as well as, in some cases, reduced adverse effects. However, it also appears that the cost of this advantage in terms of increasing risk of relapse is significant. It is particularly important to recognize that no consistent benefits of intermittent treatment have been documented in terms of social functioning or reduced risk of tardive dyskinesia. Although some individuals may be good candidates for this approach, it appears that the majority of patients would be better served with continuous treatment.

For those individuals experiencing clinically significant extrapyramidal side effects or tardive dyskinesia, the potential role of dosage-reduction strategies may be even greater. To date, no studies have focused specifically on this population, although data from outcome studies in patients with tardive dyskinesia do suggest that dosage reduction may reduce the severity of the disorder or increase the likelihood of its remission (Kane 1990).

Conclusion

A great deal of the clinical research in recent years involving antipsychotic drug treatment has focused on benefit-to-risk issues. This has been largely driven by the fact that these compounds are associated with a variety of adverse effects.

The focus on improving dosing strategies in both acute- and long-term treatment has been with the hope of reducing extrapyramidal side effects such as akinesia and akathisia as well as reducing the risk of tardive dyskinesia and tardive dystonia.

With current neuroleptic drugs, acute extrapyramidal side effects occur in as many as 50% of patients (or more, depending on assessment methodology, age, dosage, etc.), and the incidence of tardive dyskinesia is approximately 5% per year of neuroleptic exposure (Kane 1990).

The role of conventional treatment has been painstakingly established over the past three decades of clinical research in schizophrenia. However, the limitations of currently available medications are apparent to clinicians, patients, and families. The future role of these drugs will be determined by the relative merits of newer compounds. The fact that clozapine has been shown to have superior efficacy in refractory patients and reduced propensity to cause neurological side effects suggests that such advances are possible. Careful comparisons among newer and conventional neuroleptics will be critical to determine the nature and extent of the potential superiority of new compounds.

References

Carpenter WT Jr, Hanlon TE, Heinrichs DW, et al: Continuous vs. targeted medication in schizophrenic outpatients: outcome results. Am J Psychiatry 147:1138–1148, 1990

Davis JM: Overview: maintenance therapy in psychiatry, I: schizophrenia. Am J Psychiatry 132:1237–1245, 1975

Davis JM, Casper R: Antipsychotic drugs: clinical pharmacology and therapeutic use. Drugs 14:260–282, 1977

Glazer WM, Kane JM: Depot neuroleptic therapy: an underutilized treatment option. J Clin Psychiatry 53:426–433, 1992

Herz MI, Melville C: Relapse in schizophrenia. Am J Psychiatry 137:801–805, 1980

Herz MI, Glazer WM, Mostert MA, et al: Intermittent vs. maintenance medication in schizophrenia: two-year results. Arch Gen Psychiatry 48:333–339, 1991

Hogarty GE: Depot neuroleptics: the relevance of psychosocial factors. J Clin Psychiatry 45 (suppl):36–42, 1984

Hogarty GE, McEvoy JP, Munetz M, et al: Dose of fluphenazine, familial expressed emotion and outcome in schizophrenia. Arch Gen Psychiatry 45:797–805, 1988

Johnson DAW, Ludlow JM, Street K, et al: Double-blind comparison of half-dose and standard flupentixol decanoate in the maintenance treatment of stabilized outpatients with schizophrenia. Br J Psychiatry 151:634–638, 1987

Jolley AG, Hirsch SR, McRink A, et al: Trial of brief intermittent prophylaxis for selected schizophrenia outpatients: clinical outcome at one year. BMJ 298:985–990, 1989

Jolley AG, Hirsch SR, Morrison E, et al: Trial of brief intermittent prophylaxis for selected schizophrenic outpatients: clinical and social outcome at two years. BMJ 301:837–842, 1990

Kane JM: Treatment of schizophrenia. Schizophr Bull 13:133–156, 1987

Kane JM: Tardive dyskinesia. Paper presented at the 30th annual meeting of the New Clinical Drug Evaluation Unit, Key Biscayne, FL, May 1990

Kane JM, Lieberman JA: Maintenance pharmacotherapy in schizophrenia, in Psychopharmacology: The Third Generation of Progress: The Emergency of Molecular Biology and Biological Psychiatry. Edited by Meltzer HY. New York, Raven, 1987, pp 1103–1109

Kane JM, Rifkin A, Woerner M, et al: Low-dose neuroleptic treatment of outpatient schizophrenics, I: preliminary results for relapse rates. Arch Gen Psychiatry 40:893–896, 1983

Kane JM, Rifkin A, Woerner M, et al: High-dose versus low-dose strategies in the treatment of schizophrenia. Psychopharmacol Bull 21:533–537, 1985

Kane J, Honigfeld G, Singer J, et al: Clozapine for the treatment-resistant schizophrenic: a double-blind comparison with chlorpromazine. Arch Gen Psychiatry 45:789–796, 1988

Kinon B, Kane JM, Johns C, et al: Treatment of neuroleptic resistant schizophrenic relapse. Psychopharmacol Bull 29:309–314, 1993

Levinson DF, Simpson GM, Singh H, et al: Fluphenazine dose, clinical response and extrapyramidal symptoms during acute treatment. Arch Gen Psychiatry 47:761–768, 1990

Marder SR, Van Putten T, Mintz J, et al: Costs and benefits of two doses of fluphenazine. Arch Gen Psychiatry 41:1025–1029, 1984

Marder SR, Van Putten T, Mintz J, et al: Low- and conventional-dose maintenance therapy with fluphenazine decanoate: two-year outcome. Arch Gen Psychiatry 44:518–521, 1987

McEvoy JP, Hogarty G, Steingard S: Optimal dose of neuroleptic in acute schizophrenia: a controlled study of the neuroleptic threshold and higher haloperidol dose. Arch Gen Psychiatry 48:739–745, 1991

Overall JE, Gorham DR: The Brief Psychiatric Rating Scale. Psychol Rep 10:799–812, 1962

Pietzcker A, Gaebel W, Kopcke W, et al: German multicenter study on the neuroleptic long-term therapy of schizophrenic patients: preliminary report. Pharmacopsychiatry 19:161–166, 1986

Reardon GT, Rifkin A, Schwartz A, et al: Changing pattern of neuroleptic dosage over a decade. Am J Psychiatry 146:726–729, 1989

Rifkin A, Doddi S, Karagi B, et al: Dosage of haloperidol for schizophrenia. Arch Gen Psychiatry 48:166–170, 1991

Van Putten T, Marder SR, Mintz J: A controlled dose comparison of haloperidol in newly admitted schizophrenic patients. Arch Gen Psychiatry 47:754–758, 1990

CHAPTER 6

Augmenting Antipsychotic Efficacy: New Approaches

Laurence P. Karper, M.D.
John H. Krystal, M.D.

Schizophrenia is a severe and often chronic disease affecting 1%–2% of the population. Approximately 25% of patients with schizophrenia are partial responders or nonresponders to typical neuroleptic drugs. This important subgroup of patients requires alternative strategies to improve their long-term outcome (Christison et al. 1991; Pickar et al. 1991). In this chapter, we focus on the augmentation or addition of nonneuroleptic drugs to typical antipsychotic medication regimens. Although monotherapy remains the preferred treatment for neuroleptic-responsive patients, many patients who have chronic schizophrenia require polypharmacy to achieve an acceptable functional status (Wilson et al. 1985).

Evaluation

Before considering an augmentation trial, the clinician should optimize current neuroleptic medication (Kane 1989; see also Chapter 5 in this volume). Insufficient or excessive dose, noncompliance, and intolerable side effects are common factors that can result in an inadequate response to medication. When possible, injectable or decanoate preparations should be tested before concluding that an antipsychotic trial is a failure (Davis et al. 1993). Medical or neurological causes of psychosis should be evaluated before initiating augmentation. The complete evaluation of reversible causes of psychosis is beyond the scope of this chapter, but reviews of "organic" causes of psychiatric symptoms are readily available (e.g., Skuster et al. 1992).

In addition to a thorough medical and neurological evaluation, refractory patients require a psychiatric reevaluation that should focus on clarification of diagnosis and psychosocial stressors. Neuroleptics are the first choice of treatment for patients with schizophrenia. However, other patient groups may have symptoms of psychosis that require additional medications for a complete response. Patients with obsessive-compulsive disorder, bipolar disorder, posttraumatic stress disorder, borderline personality disorder, multiple personality disorder, pervasive developmental disorder, and major depression with psychotic features may receive a diagnosis of schizophrenia and may benefit from specific treatment for their disorder.

Psychosocial stressors and comorbid substance abuse can contribute to poor outcome if not addressed in a patient's treatment plan. The importance of symptom reduction in schizophrenia is underscored by longitudinal data suggesting that the long-term outcome of schizophrenia is related to the level of symptoms under optimum treatment; outcome is not related to the level of symptoms when a patient is drug free (Breier et al. 1991). Although this review focuses on the reduction of symptoms through the augmentation of typical neuroleptics, psychosocial treatments, including family treatment and rehabilitative treatments, are important strategies in the prevention of relapse (Hogarty 1993).

Although the use of an augmentation agent to treat schizophrenia can lead to symptomatic improvement, it can also increase side effects. The additional agent can cause its own side effects or can increase the toxicity of the neuroleptic. These recommendations are guidelines only. Clinicians must take into account the individual patient's history of medication use, compliance, and medical condition.

In this review, we use the framework, or algorithm, that is shown in Figure 6–1. The augmentation agents can be roughly

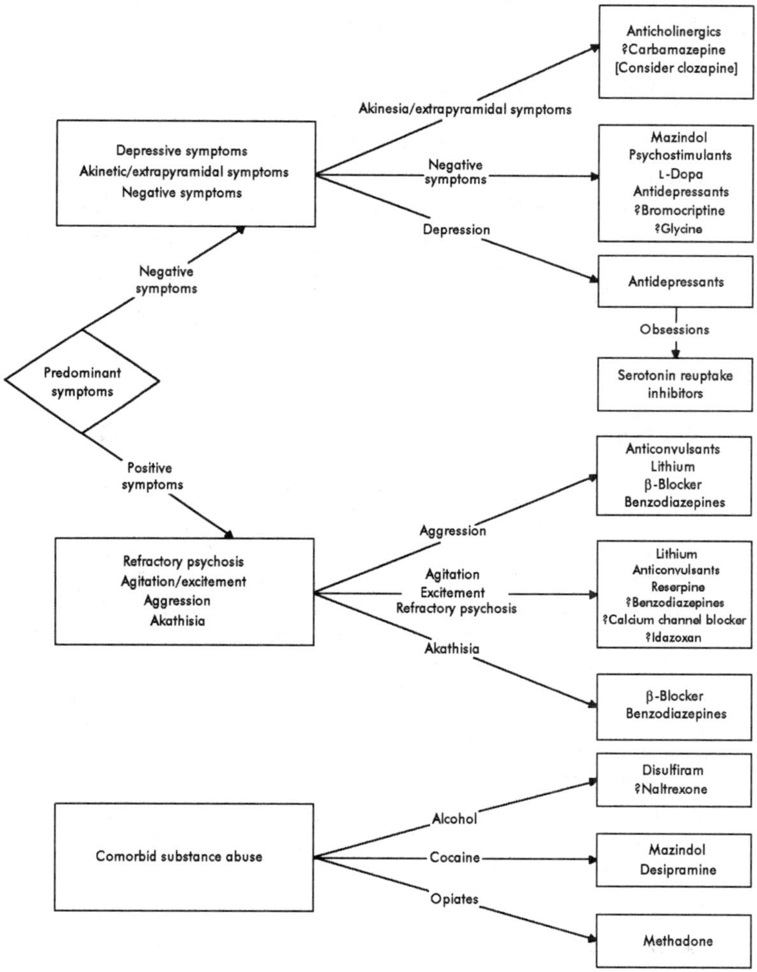

Figure 6–1. Augmentation algorithm.

divided into treatments for positive symptoms, for negative symptoms, and for comorbid substance abuse. This algorithm should be viewed as a model (not as a rigid prescription) for the augmentation of typical neuroleptic medications in the treatment of refractory schizophrenia.

Positive Symptom Treatment

Positive symptoms such as paranoia, hallucinations, thought disorder, hostility, agitation, and excitement are the most responsive to typical neuroleptic treatment. When a patient does not respond adequately to neuroleptics, an augmentation agent can be tried. A distinction can further be made between aggression (which may occur when a patient is not psychotic) and refractory psychosis (which may be associated with agitation and excitement). In addition, akathisia can be mistaken for psychosis.

Lithium

Case Example

Mr. A, a 35-year-old black veteran with chronic paranoid schizophrenia, was admitted for exacerbation of psychosis characterized by agitation and response to internal stimuli (cursing out loud almost continuously). After 4 weeks of haloperidol elixir 20 mg, Mr. A continued to curse at imaginary people and refused to participate in ward activities. The patient exhibited no specific mood symptoms, but he was quite irritable. Medical evaluation was noncontributory. The patient refused to cooperate with family meetings to assess his living situation. Lithium carbonate was begun at 300 mg bid and increased to 300 mg tid, with a blood level of 0.8 mEq/L. He developed a mild postural tremor. After 2 weeks, Mr. A continued to express some delusions but was no longer overtly hallucinating or hostile and was able to participate in ward activities and discharge planning.

Studies of Lithium Treatment of Psychosis

Lithium carbonate is the first-line treatment for bipolar disorder (Schou 1989). However, lithium has also been used to treat patients with schizophrenia since its introduction into clinical use (Schulz et al. 1990). Lithium is the drug that has been studied most often as a strategy for augmenting neuroleptic response in patients with psychosis. Studies of the efficacy of lithium in comparison to chlorpromazine for acutely ill patients with psychotic mood disorders were disappointing (Braden et al. 1982; Prien et al. 1972; Shopsin et al. 1971). These studies examined short-term treatment with lithium alone and found that chlorpromazine was more effective in reducing psychosis particularly in hostile or "highly active" patients. Studies that compared lithium with placebo added to neuroleptics in the treatment of schizophrenia and schizoaffective disorder found that lithium treatment produced improvements in both mood and psychosis (Biederman et al. 1979; Carmen et al. 1981; Growe et al. 1979; Lerner et al. 1988; Small et al. 1975). Lithium may be particularly helpful in patients with psychotic excitement (Growe et al. 1979), depressive symptoms (Lerner et al. 1988), and better interepisode functioning (Biederman et al. 1979); chronically ill, neuroleptic-refractory patients also can improve significantly (Small et al. 1975). Lithium can reduce psychosis even in patients who have no apparent mood symptoms (Alexander et al. 1979; Zemlen et al. 1984). In addition to the antimanic and antipsychotic properties of lithium, it has also been used to treat aggression in psychotic (Tupin et al. 1973) as well as in nonpsychotic populations (Sheard et al. 1976). The mechanism of action of lithium is unknown, but its effects on serotonin (Eichelman 1988) or dopamine metabolism (Bowers et al. 1992) may result in decreased hostility or improved response to neuroleptics.

Side Effects and Usage

Lithium can lower the seizure threshold and can therefore cause seizures when used in conjunction with neuroleptics. Lithium should be used cautiously in patients with epilepsy or organic brain syndromes. Lithium alone (Prakash et al. 1982a; Rifkin et al. 1973) or in combination with haloperidol may cause delirium even at therapeutic doses (Cohen and Cohen 1974). Acutely ill patients may be at a higher risk for developing neurotoxicity (Spring and Frankel 1981). Confusion, increased extrapyramidal symptoms, cerebellar signs, and fever are typical symptoms and signs of lithium toxicity (Prakash et al. 1982b). Even though treatment with lithium and haloperidol (and other neuroleptics) may result in toxicity, two retrospective studies including more than 500 patients found that long-term treatment with lithium and neuroleptics was well tolerated (Baastrup et al. 1976; Goldney and Spence 1986).

Common side effects are fine postural tremor that is particularly noticeable in the fingers (responsive to propranolol but not to anticholinergic agents), coarse intention tremor (may be an early sign of toxicity), nausea, sedation, diarrhea, nephrogenic diabetes insipidus, and hypothyroidism. In addition, lithium may increase parkinsonian side effects when used in combination with neuroleptics (Addonizio et al. 1988). Relative contraindications to the use of lithium are renal, thyroid, and cardiovascular disease (especially atrioventricular conduction disturbances). During treatment with lithium, renal and thyroid function must be checked periodically. Lithium is usually initiated at 300–900 mg/day in 2–3 divided doses. Initially, lithium levels should be followed closely. The level should be titrated to between 0.5 and 1.0 mEq/L as tolerated. To reduce side effects when lithium augmentation is begun, it may be necessary to reduce neuroleptic dosages by 10%–25%.

Anticonvulsants: Carbamazepine and Valproic Acid

Theoretical Background

Carbamazepine and valproic acid are the anticonvulsants most often studied as augmentation agents. The use of other anticonvulsants in the treatment of schizophrenia is beyond the scope of this review. Anticonvulsant treatment of psychiatric disorders has been given impetus by the beneficial psychotropic effects of carbamazepine seen in patients treated for epilepsy (Dalby 1971; Dodrill and Troupin 1977). Clinical reports of psychiatric syndromes occurring in patients with temporal lobe epilepsy (Slater and Beard 1963; Waxman and Geschwind 1974, 1975) led to preclinical research on the behavioral effects of limbic kindling (Adamec and Stark-Adamec 1983; Post et al. 1984; Stevens and Livermore 1978). These investigations further supported the use of anticonvulsants that inhibit limbic kindling in psychiatric disorders. However, the mechanism of action of carbamazepine and valproic acid in the treatment of the positive symptoms of schizophrenia is unclear.

Carbamazepine

The initial reports of the use of carbamazepine in psychiatric patients focused on psychotic patients with aggression or abnormal electroencephalograms. These studies (Hakola and Laulumaa 1982; Luchins 1983; Neppe 1983) demonstrated that carbamazepine may be effective in reducing aggressive behavior and psychotic symptoms. In a single-blind study, Herrera et al. (1987) found carbamazepine to be useful as an adjunctive treatment. In this study, carbamazepine reduced social withdrawal, depression, and anxiety in treatment-resistant patients with schizophrenia. Two double-blind, placebo-controlled trials (Klein et al. 1984; Okuma et al. 1989) of the addition of carbamazepine to neuroleptics in patients with schizophrenia demonstrated that carbamazepine efficacy was superior to placebo in the reduction of psychotic symptoms, especially in excited or hostile patients. Carbamazepine in the reduction in psychotic symptoms, however, was not superior to placebo in two other double-blind, placebo-controlled trials of carbamazepine augmentation of neuroleptics (Dose et al. 1987; Kidron et al. 1985). The Dose et al. study did report, however, that the carbamazepine-treated patients had fewer side effects and required less neuroleptic medication. Carbamazepine has not been shown to be an effective single treatment for schizophrenia (W. T. Carpenter et al. 1991; Sramek et al. 1988). Carbamazepine may be effective for patients with refractory hallucinations and a history of hallucinogen abuse (Scher and Neppe 1989).

Although carbamazepine is usually well tolerated, significant side effects can occur, including diplopia, ataxia, gastrointestinal upset, rash, agranulocytosis, cardiac arrhythmias, and hepatic toxicity. Whereas short-term treatment with carbamazepine is usually well tolerated, long-term treatment may be compromised by hematological and hepatic side effects (Frankenburg et al. 1988). Carbamazepine can also cause hyponatremia (Henry et al. 1977), which is particularly problematic in psychotic patients with polydipsia (Jose and Perez-Cruet 1979). Abnormally low sodium levels before treatment and carbamazepine responsiveness may be risk factors for carbamazepine-induced hyponatremia (Uhde and Post 1983). The addition of lithium to carbamazepine may reduce carbamazepine-induced hyponatremia (Vieweg et al. 1987). Carbamazepine can be initiated at 200 mg bid and titrated to a level of 8–12 mg/L (Post et al. 1989). Carbamazepine can reduce the blood level of haloperidol as a result of hepatic enzyme induction (Jann et al. 1985), and this reduction in neuroleptic blood levels may explain why some patients worsen on carbamazepine (E. M. Kahn et al. 1990; Pickar et al. 1991). Because of carbamazepine's autoinduction of hepatic enzymes, blood levels must be monitored closely for several months after initiating therapy. Because the blood level of carbamazepine will drop several weeks after achieving an initial steady state, relapse may occur related to a withdrawal phenomenon (Heh et al. 1988). When carbamazepine is discontinued, neuroleptic blood levels may rise and result in increased extrapyramidal side effects (Jann et al. 1989).

Valproic Acid

In their review of the effectiveness of valproic acid in the treatment of schizophrenia, McElroy and co-workers (1989) reported that 30% of patients appeared to benefit. Although several reports have supported the use of valproic acid in patients with schizophrenia (Linnoila et al. 1976; Nagao et al. 1979; VanValkenburg et al. 1990; Wassef et al. 1989), the only double-blind trial with operationalized diagnostic criteria did not find it useful as an adjunctive agent (Ko et al. 1985). Based on the success of valproic acid in the treatment of mania, it may be expected to be particularly useful in the treatment of excited psychotic states and schizoaffective disorder (McElroy et al. 1989; Pope et al. 1991). Valproic acid appears to be less likely than carbamazepine to cause hyponatremia and may be especially useful in patients who have psychosis and polydipsia that is refractory to neuroleptic treatment (Karper et al. 1992).

At our center, valproic acid has been useful when added to either typical neuroleptics or clozapine for the treatment of refractory psychosis. Valproic acid can be useful in the treatment of a diverse group of clinical situations, including dementia with agitation, epilepsy with comorbid psychosis, and schizophrenia with predominant excitement. Two reports of the efficacy of valproic acid in patients who have a history of head injury or organic mental disorders are encouraging (D. Kahn et al. 1988; Pope et al. 1988) given the difficulty in treating this population. Major side effects of valproic acid include sedation, coarse postural and intention tremor (treatable with propranolol), liver function abnormalities and hepatitis (rarely severe hepatotoxicity), gastrointestinal upset, and platelet dysfunction. Several patients have experienced delirium while receiving therapeutic levels of valproic acid, and some patients have had high serum levels of ammonia. Valproic acid can be started at 250 mg bid and titrated to a level of 80–100 μg/ml. Some patients who have abdominal complaints may tolerate divalproex sodium, an enteric-coated form of valproic acid.

Indications for the Use of Anticonvulsants

Carbamazepine and valproic acid are useful in the treatment of psychosis and comorbid organic syndromes when an anticonvulsant is needed. In patients who have failed conventional treatment and who have persistent hostility or excitement, carbamazepine (or as a second-line agent, valproic acid) can be used instead of or in addition to lithium. Patients we have treated who required neuroleptics, lithium, and anticonvulsants tolerated the combination well; however, side effects, particularly tremor, may prove difficult to alleviate. In general, the gains from anticonvulsant treatment of psychotic symptoms may be modest. However, because the anticonvulsants (especially carbamazepine) may reduce hostility and violent behavior, even modest improvements in symptoms may allow the patient to be maintained in a less restrictive inpatient or outpatient setting. The literature on the use of anticonvulsants in schizophrenia is small, but it does suggest that these agents have a place in the treatment of a subgroup of patients with schizophrenia.

β-*Blockers*

Treatment of Psychosis With β-Blockers

β-Adrenergic receptor antagonists—β-blockers—are used primarily in the treatment of hypertension and cardiovascular disease. Propranolol, pindolol, metoprolol, and nadolol are drugs of this class that have been studied in the treatment of schizophrenia, akathisia, and aggression. Propranolol has been the most studied of these agents in the treatment of schizophrenia. Propranolol is frequently used in the treatment of aggression in patients with organic mental disorders (Yudofsky et al. 1981).

The results of double-blind, placebo-controlled studies of propranolol have not shown a consistent antipsychotic effect alone or in addition to neuroleptics (Christison et al. 1991). It is difficult to compare these studies because each used a different dose of propranolol and evaluated populations that varied with regard to chronicity. There were no consistent predictors of response to propranolol (Lindstrom and Persson 1980; Myers et al. 1981; Peet et al. 1981a; Pugh et al. 1983; Yorkston et al. 1981). One explanation for the inconsistent results in these studies is that the improvement found is related not to a specific antipsychotic effect of propranolol but instead to a reduction in akathisia (Lipinski et al. 1988). Akathisia, a subjective sense of anxiety or uneasiness often associated with "marching in place," is a side effect caused by neuroleptic medications. This side effect can be mistaken for worsening psychosis, can lead to clinical deterioration, and rarely precipitates violent (Crowner et al. 1990) or even suicidal behavior (Drake and Erhrlich 1985). Propranolol is an effective treatment for neuroleptic-induced akathisia and should be tried in patients who cannot tolerate neuroleptics because of akathisia (Lipinski et al. 1984). β-Blockers also appear to be effective for some patients who have schizophrenia with impulsivity or aggression (Ratey et al. 1992; Sorgi et al. 1986).

Side Effects and Usage

β-Blockers should be used with caution in patients with a history of cardiovascular or peripheral vascular disease, asthma or chronic lung disease, or diabetes. The main side effects of β-blockers are hypotension and bradycardia. In patients at risk for hypotension or bradycardia (elderly or dehydrated patients), begin with a 20-mg test dose of propranolol, and, if tolerated, the dose may be increased by 20 mg/day every 3 days (J. M. Silver et al. 1990). In individuals unlikely to experience the cardiovascular side effects of β-blockers, start propranolol at 20 mg twice a day and increase by 60 mg/day every 3 days. Do not administer propranolol if the heart rate is below 50 beats/minute or if the systolic blood pressure is less than 90 mm Hg. Discontinue propranolol (taper if it is at a high dose to avoid rebound hypertension and obtain medical consultation) if ataxia, dizziness, or wheezing occurs. Decreases in akathisia may be seen in 1–3 days with 30–80 mg/day of propranolol (Lipinski et al. 1984); however, doses as high as 800 mg/day for 8 weeks may be required for its antiaggressive efficacy (J. M. Silver et al. 1990). Propranolol is relatively contraindicated in patients with a history of a mood disorder because it may exacerbate or cause depression. Propranolol can cause toxic reactions in patients treated with chlorpromazine (Thorazine) (Miller and Rampling 1982; Peet et al. 1981b) and thioridazine (Greendyke and Kanter 1987) because propranolol increases antipsychotic blood levels. In summary, β-blockers appear to have a modest effect on psychotic symptoms in conjunction with antipsychotics but may have a significant clinical effect in patients with violent outbursts or akathisia.

Reserpine

Reserpine, a rauwolfia alkaloid, is a presynaptic depleter of catecholamine and serotonin stores in the brain. Reserpine is used primarily as an antihypertensive agent, although reports of its use in the treatment of insanity date back to ancient Hindu Ayurvedic texts (Weiner 1985). Reserpine was used to treat psychosis before the introduction of neuroleptics in the 1950s (Christison et al. 1991). Studies of the efficacy of reserpine found that it reduced psychotic symptoms as well as hostility (Finn et al. 1955; Gore et al. 1957). The addition of reserpine to neuroleptics and lithium may improve antipsychotic response, especially in patients with schizoaffective or bipolar disorder (Berlant 1986). A case report suggested that the combination of diazepam and reserpine 2 mg/day was effective in a patient refractory to neuroleptics with a history of tardive dyskinesia (Bacher et al. 1989). Reserpine may be particularly useful in the treatment of patients with severe tardive dyskinesia because it decreases dyskinesias and rarely causes tardive dyskinesia (Task Force on Tardive Dyskinesia 1992).

When chlorpromazine became available, reserpine use dwindled because of its side effects, including hypotension, depression, asthma, exacerbation of peptic ulcer, and extrapyramidal side effects. Doses of 8–12 mg/day (1–5 mg/day with neuroleptics) appear to achieve the best response. Patients should be started gradually and the dose increased by 0.25 mg/week to reduce side effects. A trial of reserpine should last 5–7 weeks (Christison et al. 1991).

Benzodiazepines

Benzodiazepines with or without neuroleptics are clearly indicated for the acute treatment of agitation and excitement in an acute relapse of schizophrenia (Garza-Trevino et al. 1989; Salzman et al. 1986). Adjunctive benzodiazepines for the maintenance treatment of schizophrenia can be of some help in one-third to one-half of patients (for review, see Wolkowitz and Pickar 1991; Wolkowitz et al. 1992; see also Chapter 8 in this volume). Subgroups of patients with akathisia, anxiety, or agitation may benefit from the addition of a benzodiazepine (Wolkowitz and Pickar 1991). A particular difficulty with the use of benzodiazepines is their abuse potential and the development of tolerance. The chronic use of benzodiazepines should be reserved for patients who clearly benefit from their effects and who do not abuse them. The major side effects of the benzodiazepines are sedation, ataxia, memory disturbance, and confusion. Benzodiazepines with active metabolites, such as diazepam, should be avoided in the elderly or in patients with liver disease. Lorazepam is an intermediate-acting benzodiazepine without active metabolites that is frequently used to control acute psychotic agitation and can be used in the treatment of schizophrenia when patients have prominent anxiety symptoms or akathisia refractory to propranolol treatment.

Calcium Channel Blockers

Calcium channel blockers are medications used in the treatment of cardiovascular disease. Verapamil, nifedipine, and diltiazem have been studied in the treatment of psychosis and tardive dyskinesia (Bartko et al. 1991; Duncan et al. 1990; Pickar et al. 1987; Reiter et al. 1989; Ross et al. 1987; Stedman et al. 1991; Suddath et al. 1991). These agents may produce modest decreases in tardive dyskinesia and psychotic symptoms but should be used with caution because verapamil has led to increased hostility in some patients (Pickar et al. 1987). The mechanism of action of these agents may be through blockade of the dopamine system or pharmacokinetic interactions with neuroleptics (Duncan et al. 1990; Stedman et al. 1991). Further studies are needed to better assess the utility of these agents.

Noradrenergic Agents

Idazoxan, a potent and selective α_2-adrenergic-receptor antagonist, is a drug that increases noradrenergic function. Idazoxan has been investigated in the treatment of schizophrenia because clozapine also possesses α_2-adrenergic-receptor antagonism. Preliminary work has suggested that idazoxan reduces psychotic symptoms in some patients with schizophrenia (Litman et al. 1992). Idazoxan (and possibly yohimbine, another α_2-adrenergic-receptor antagonist) may prove to be quite helpful in the treatment of patients with schizophrenia.

Negative Symptom Treatment

Negative symptoms frequently do not respond to neuroleptic treatment as well as positive symptoms do. Negative symptoms may be chronic and are characterized by a lack of motivation, energy, speech, affect, and interest as well as by the presence of concrete thought. These symptoms are less dramatic than positive symptoms, but they can be quite disabling. It is important to try to distinguish negative symptoms from subtle extrapyramidal symptoms such as akinesia/bradykinesia, masked facies, and rigidity. A trial of an anticholinergic medication is indicated when extrapyramidal side effects impair functioning. Also, use of clozapine or a low-potency neuroleptic should be considered when parkinsonian side effects are not tolerated.

Dopaminergic Agents

Theoretical Background

The dopamine hypothesis of schizophrenia was based in part on the observation that medications that increase dopamine levels in the brain, such as amphetamine and L-dopa, can cause a paranoid psychosis indistinguishable from schizophrenia. As the dopamine hypothesis was refined, efforts were made to understand both positive and negative symptoms in terms of either increased or decreased dopamine function in the brain. Further support for this hypothesis came from data suggesting that negative symptoms were reduced in some patients with schizophrenia after an acute amphetamine challenge (e.g., Goldberg et al. 1991). This led investigators to evaluate the effect of dopaminergic medications on negative symptoms in stable medicated patients with schizophrenia.

Treatment of Schizophrenia With Dopaminergic Agents

L-Dopa and the psychostimulants (amphetamine, methylphenidate, and pemoline) increase the synthesis and release of dopamine in the brain and have been studied in patients with schizophrenia (Alpert et al. 1978; Angrist et al. 1980; M. D. Carpenter et al. 1992; Cesarec and Nyman 1985; Gerlach and Luhdorf 1975; for a review of the use of psychostimulants in psychiatry, see Chiarello and Cole 1987). In general, these studies support the view that these agents can be used cautiously in patients with schizophrenia, with resulting modest improvements in negative symptoms. These agents do carry the risk of increasing positive symptoms. The psychostimulants can increase blood pressure and heart rate and are therefore contraindicated in patients with significant coronary artery disease or hypertension. In addition, because amphetamine has significant abuse potential, it should be prescribed with care to patients who are at risk for drug abuse.

Bromocriptine, a potent dopaminergic agonist, has reduced positive and negative symptoms of schizophrenia in a pilot study using 2.5 mg/day in addition to neuroleptics (Wolf et al. 1992). Higher doses may lead to clinical deterioration (Tamminga and Schaffer 1979). Bromocriptine is often used in patients with Parkinson's disease, but it has not been studied extensively in patients with schizophrenia and could conceivably worsen psychosis, especially at high doses.

Mazindol is a dopamine reuptake inhibitor that has been used to treat negative symptoms in patients with schizophrenia (Seibyl et al. 1992b). Mazindol at doses of 1–3 mg/day has been well tolerated with only occasional side effects of mild insomnia and anorexia. Patients have had clinically significant improvements in their daily functioning, which allows them to engage in rehabilitative activities. For patients seeking help with negative symptoms, mazindol is a useful augmentation strategy with few of the side effects of L-dopa or psychostimulants.

Serotonin-Receptor Antagonists

Clozapine and risperidone are potent serotonin-receptor antagonists. These two drugs are effective in reducing symptoms of schizophrenia and are less likely than typical neuroleptics to cause extrapyramidal side effects. The fact that the combination of serotonin- and dopamine-receptor blockade could account for the improved efficacy of atypical neuroleptics led to the use of specific serotonin-receptor blockers to treat schizophrenia. Ritanserin (Gelders 1989) and amperozide (Axelsson et al. 1991)—serotonin$_2$ (5-HT$_2$) receptor blockers—have been used with neuroleptics to treat schizophrenia with some reduction in symptoms. These agents appeared to be helpful in the treatment of negative symptoms. Cyproheptadine, a 5-HT$_2$-receptor antagonist with anticholinergic and antihistaminic properties, used as an augmentation agent with typical neuroleptics has reduced psychotic symptoms in some refractory patients (H. Silver et al. 1989). However, a double-blind, placebo-controlled study of cyproheptadine in patients with chronic schizophrenia showed no benefit (H. Silver et al. 1991). One report found that zacopride, a 5-HT$_3$-receptor blocker, was not helpful as a sole agent in the treatment of schizophrenia (Newcomer et al. 1992); however, it may prove to have some use as an augmentation agent. Preliminary evidence suggests that specific serotonin blockers may be useful in some patients, but further definition of the benefits of these agents awaits further study.

Glycine

N-methyl-D-aspartate (NMDA)-receptor antagonists such as phencyclidine and ketamine produce a clinical picture similar to that of psychosis (for a review, see Javitt and Zukin 1991). These drugs produce both positive and negative symptoms of schizophrenia (Krystal et al. 1994). Large oral doses of glycine (5–25 g/day) have been used to increase NMDA-receptor function in schizophrenia with some encouraging results (Costa et al. 1990; Nussenzveig et al. 1992; Waziri 1988). Current research is focusing on developing drugs that increase NMDA neurotransmission and reliably cross the blood-brain barrier without excessive side effects. Milacemide, an acylated prodrug of glycine that crosses the blood-brain barrier, has not demonstrated efficacy in high or low doses (Rosse et al. 1991). D-Cycloserine, a partial agonist at the glycine site of the NMDA receptor, is an antibiotic that crosses the blood-brain barrier. It has been used to reverse scopolamine dementia (Jones et al. 1991), and studies are under way to investigate its use in schizophrenia.

Antidepressants

Tricyclic Antidepressants

Tricyclic antidepressants can reduce depressive and negative symptoms when used to treat depression in patients with schizophrenia (Siris et al. 1987, 1991; for a review, see Siris 1990; see also Chapter 10 in this volume). The patients who benefit most are those who have a clear depression and whose side effects such as neuroleptic-induced akinesia have been vigorously treated. Patients stabilized on neuroleptics before the addition of an antidepressant often tolerate antidepressants without increases in psychotic symptoms. Actively psychotic patients may experience increases in psychotic symptoms when an antidepressant is added (Kramer et al. 1989). When positive psychotic symptoms recur or worsen after a trial of an antidepressant has begun, an increase in neuroleptic dose may be helpful (Siris 1990).

Monoamine Oxidase Inhibitors (MAOIs)

Another approach to the treatment of negative symptoms is to increase dopamine function by blocking the degradation of dopamine with the use of MAOIs (Bucci 1987). Selegiline, a specific MAOI-B that does not require the use of dietary restrictions, may have some efficacy in reducing negative symptoms (Bodkin et al. 1992; Perenyi et al. 1992).

Serotonin Reuptake Inhibitors

Fluoxetine, fluvoxamine, and clomipramine are serotonin reuptake inhibitors that have been used in the treatment of schizophrenia (Berman et al. 1993; Goff et al. 1990; Goldman and Janecek 1990; Hwang et al. 1993; H. Silver and Nassar 1992). These agents improved negative symptoms (H. Silver and Nassar 1992), global functioning (Goldman and Janecek 1990), positive and negative symptoms in nondepressed patients (Goff et al. 1990), and obsessive-compulsive symptoms (Berman et al. 1993; Hwang et al. 1993) in some patients with schizophrenia. Although these studies suggested that these agents can produce modest improvements in symptoms, some patients may deteriorate after receiving a serotonin reuptake inhibitor (Lindenmayer et al. 1990). Most patients will tolerate fluoxetine without experiencing increased extrapyramidal symptoms; however, fluoxetine can increase neuroleptic blood levels by 20% and may lead to akathisia (Goff et al. 1991). These results are clearly preliminary, but they do suggest a role for serotonin reuptake inhibitors in schizophrenia, especially for the reduction of obsessive symptoms.

Comorbid Substance Abuse

Antidipsotropic Agents: Disulfiram and Naltrexone

Disulfiram is a medication that produces toxic side effects when combined with alcohol (Kosten and Kosten 1991). It has been used extensively in the treatment of alcoholism, but concerns have been raised about its use in schizophrenia because it may exacerbate psychosis (Macklin et al. 1953). We have found this medication to be useful in the treatment of schizophrenia when combined with clozapine in a stable patient (Brenner et al. 1994). Because lethal side effects are possible when patients drink alcohol while taking disulfiram, it must be used with caution. Patients who are motivated, have insight into their illness, and have adequate psychosocial supports are good candidates for this treatment. Naltrexone is an opiate antagonist that has been shown to reduce relapse rates in alcoholic patients (O'Malley et al. 1992); it is currently being investigated in the treatment of schizophrenia with comorbid alcohol abuse.

Cocaine Abuse

Few controlled studies have examined the treatment of cocaine abuse in patients with schizophrenia. With the advent of the epidemic of "crack" cocaine use, the treatment of patients with schizophrenia who abuse cocaine has become more of a challenge. Desipramine (Ziedonis et al. 1992) and mazindol (Johnson et al.

1992; Seibyl et al. 1992a) have some promise in this area. In the Ziedonis et al. study, patients with schizophrenia who abused cocaine were treated with desipramine to reduce their use of cocaine in the context of a specific dual-diagnosis treatment program. At our center, we utilize mazindol in the context of a specially designed dual-diagnosis group to provide extra support to this population.

Opiate Dependence

Methadone can be used to treat opiate dependence in patients with schizophrenia. Two reports suggest that methadone can reduce psychotic symptoms in patients with schizophrenia (Brizer et al. 1985; Feinberg and Hartman 1991). Methadone is usually given in the context of a structured program in which it can be used in the treatment of people who abuse intravenous heroin.

Summary and Recommendations

No "one size fits all" prescription can be articulated for the augmentation treatment of refractory schizophrenia. Refractory patients usually have complicated combinations of biological, environmental, and psychosocial vulnerabilities that lead to neuroleptic-resistant psychosis. Before beginning a trial of an augmentation agent, a target symptom or symptom cluster must be chosen to become the focus of treatment. Then the target symptom can be followed with relevant symptom rating scales or objective behavioral measures to document efficacy. Frequently, successful trials produce only modest reductions in symptomatology (10%–20%). Based on the incremental benefit of these agents, the risks and benefits of their use must be clearly documented. Even modest reductions in well-chosen target symptoms can increase the quality of life for these severely ill patients. Successful trials often target behaviors or symptoms that patients themselves find distressing, although this is not always possible because of the lack of insight that is endemic to this population.

The single most important decision in augmentation is the nature of the predominant symptoms to be treated. For positive symptoms, lithium, carbamazepine, and valproic acid are the first-line agents. Benzodiazepines and β-blockers are often quite successful in reducing akathisia and can be useful in the reduction of aggression. Negative symptom treatments are not as well studied, but, in our institution, mazindol is the first-line agent under investigation. For depressed patients without active psychotic symptoms, an antidepressant appears to be a reasonable choice even though some patients may have psychotic exacerbations. Dopaminergic agents such as L-dopa, amphetamine, and bromocriptine can be used to treat negative symptoms, but caution is necessary given the side effects and particularly the psychotogenic effects of these drugs. Comorbid substance use can be treated with desipramine or mazindol for cocaine abuse and disulfiram or possibly naltrexone for alcoholism. The other drugs discussed in this chapter—calcium channel blockers, glycine, reserpine, serotonin-receptor antagonists, MAOIs, and noradrenergic agents—may have a future role in the routine armamentarium of refractory schizophrenia when predictors for response are better delineated.

References

Adamec RE, Stark-Adamec C: Limbic kindling and animal behavior—implications for human psychopathology associated with complex partial seizures. Biol Psychiatry 18:269–293, 1983

Addonizio G, Roth SD, Stokes PE, Stoll PM: Increased extrapyramidal symptoms with addition of lithium to neuroleptics. J Nerv Ment Dis 176:682–685, 1988

Alexander PE, Van Kammen DP, Bunney WE: Antipsychotic effects of lithium in schizophrenia. Am J Psychiatry 136:283–287, 1979

Alpert M, Friedhoff AJ, Marcos LR, et al: Paradoxical reaction to L-dopa in schizophrenic patients. Am J Psychiatry 135:1329–1332, 1978

Angrist B, Rotrosen J, Gershon S: Differential effects of amphetamine and neuroleptics on negative vs. positive symptoms in schizophrenia. Psychopharmacology 72:17–19, 1980

Axelsson R, Nilsson A, Christensson E, et al: Effects of amperozide in schizophrenia: an open study of a potent 5-HT_2 receptor antagonist. Psychopharmacology 104:287–292, 1991

Baastrup PC, Hollnagel P, Sorensen R, et al: Adverse reactions in treatment with lithium carbonate and haloperidol. JAMA 236:2645–2646, 1976

Bacher NM, Field PB, Elkashef A: Possible enhancing effects of diazepam with reserpine in a chronic schizophrenic patient with tardive dyskinesia (letter). J Clin Psychopharmacol 9:312, 1989

Bartko G, Horvath S, Zador G, et al: Effects of adjunctive verapamil administration in chronic schizophrenic patients. Prog Neuropsychopharmacol Biol Psychiatry 15:343–349, 1991

Berlant JL: Neuroleptics and reserpine in refractory psychoses. J Clin Psychopharmacol 6:180–184, 1986

Berman I, Sapers BL, Chang HHJ, et al: Adjunctive clomipramine in obsessive schizophrenia (NR11), in New Research Program and Abstracts: American Psychiatric Association 146th Annual Meeting, San Francisco, CA, May 22–27, 1993, p 61

Biederman J, Lerner Y, Belmaker RH: Combination of lithium carbonate and haloperidol in schizoaffective disorder: a controlled study. Arch Gen Psychiatry 36:327–333, 1979

Bodkin A, Cannon S, Cohen B, et al: Selegiline treatment of negative symptoms of schizophrenia and schizoaffective disorder. Abstracts of panels and posters presented at the 31st annual meeting of the American College of Neuropsychopharmacology, San Juan, Puerto Rico, December 14–18, 1992

Bowers MB Jr, Mazure CM, Nelson JC, et al: Lithium in combination with perphenazine: effect on plasma monoamine metabolites. Biol Psychiatry 32:1102–1107, 1992

Braden W, Fink EB, Qualls CB, et al: Lithium and chlorpromazine in psychotic inpatients. Psychiatry Res 7:69–81, 1982

Breier A, Schreiber JL, Dyer J, et al: National Institute of Mental Health longitudinal study of chronic schizophrenia: prognosis and prediction of outcome. Arch Gen Psychiatry 48:239–246, 1991

Brenner LM, Karper LP, Krystal JH: Short-term use of disulfiram with clozapine (letter). J Clin Psychopharmacol 14:213–215, 1994

Brizer DA, Hartman N, Sweeney J, et al: Effect of methadone plus neuroleptics on treatment-resistant chronic paranoid schizophrenia. Am J Psychiatry 142:1106–1107, 1985

Bucci L: The negative symptoms of schizophrenia and the monoamine oxidase inhibitors. Psychopharmacology (Berl) 91:104–108, 1987

Carmen JS, Bigelow LB, Wyatt RJ: Lithium combined with neuroleptics in chronic schizophrenic and schizoaffective patients. J Clin Psychiatry 42:124–128, 1981

Carpenter MD, Winsberg BG, Camus LA: Methylphenidate augmentation therapy in schizophrenia. J Clin Psychopharmacol 12:273–275, 1992

Carpenter WT Jr, Kurz R, Kirkpatrick B, et al: Carbamazepine maintenance treatment in outpatient schizophrenics. Arch Gen Psychiatry 48:69–72, 1991

Cesarec Z, Nyman AK: Differential effects to amphetamine in schizophrenia. Acta Psychiatr Scand 71:523–538, 1985

Chiarello RJ, Cole JO: The use of psychostimulants in general psychiatry: a reconsideration. Arch Gen Psychiatry 44:286–295, 1987

Christison GW, Kirch DG, Wyatt RJ: When symptoms persist: choosing among alternative somatic treatments for schizophrenia. Schizophr Bull 17:217–245, 1991

Cohen WJ, Cohen NH: Lithium carbonate, haloperidol, and irreversible brain damage. JAMA 230:1283–1287, 1974

Costa J, Khaled E, Sramek J, et al: An open trial of glycine as an adjunct to neuroleptics in chronic treatment-refractory schizophrenics. J Clin Psychopharmacol 10:71–72, 1990

Crowner ML, Douyon R, Convit A, et al: Akathisia and violence. Psychopharmacol Bull 26:115–117, 1990

Dalby MA: Antiepileptic and psychotropic effect of carbamazepine (Tegretol) in the treatment of psychomotor epilepsy. Epilepsia 12:325–334, 1971

Davis JM, Kane JM, Marder SR, et al: Dose response of prophylactic antipsychotics. J Clin Psychiatry 54 (suppl 3):24–30, 1993

Dodrill CB, Troupin AS: Psychotropic effects of carbamazepine in epilepsy: a double-blind comparison with phenytoin. Neurology 27:1023–1028, 1977

Dose M, Apelt S, Emrich HM: Carbamazepine as an adjunct of antipsychotic therapy. Psychiatry Res 22:303–310, 1987

Drake RE, Erhrlich J: Suicide attempts associated with akathisia. Am J Psychiatry 142:499–501, 1985

Duncan E, Adler L, Angrist B, et al: Nifedipine in the treatment of tardive dyskinesia. J Clin Psychopharmacol 10:414–416, 1990

Eichelman B: Toward a rational pharmacotherapy for aggressive and violent behavior. Hosp Community Psychiatry 39:31–39, 1988

Feinberg DT, Hartman N: Methadone and schizophrenia. Am J Psychiatry 148:1750–1751, 1991

Finn MHP, Nadolksi F, Guy W, et al: Clinical, psychological and myoneural changes in psychotic patients under oral Serpasil medication. J Nerv Ment Dis 122:458–462, 1955

Frankenburg FR, Tohen M, Cohen BM, et al: Long-term response to carbamazepine: a retrospective study. J Clin Psychopharmacol 8:130–132, 1988

Garza-Trevino ES, Hollister LE, Overall JE, et al: Efficacy of combinations of intramuscular antipsychotics and sedative-hypnotics for control of psychotic agitation. Am J Psychiatry 146:1598–1601, 1989

Gelders YG: Thymosthenic agents, a novel approach in the treatment of schizophrenia. Br J Psychiatry 155 (suppl 5):33–36, 1989

Gerlach J, Luhdorf K: The effect of L-dopa on young patients with simple schizophrenia, treated with neuroleptic drugs. Psychopharmacologia 44:105–110, 1975

Goff DC, Brotman AW, Waites M, et al: Trial of fluoxetine added to neuroleptics for treatment-resistant schizophrenic patients. Am J Psychiatry 147:492–494, 1990

Goff DC, Midha KK, Brotman AW, et al: Elevation of plasma concentrations of haloperidol after the addition of fluoxetine. Am J Psychiatry 148:790–792, 1991

Goldberg TE, Bigelow LB, Weinberger DR, et al: Cognitive and behavioral effects of the coadministration of dextroamphetamine and haloperidol in schizophrenia. Am J Psychiatry 148:78–84, 1991

Goldman MB, Janecek HM: Adjunctive fluoxetine improves global function in chronic schizophrenia. J Neuropsychiatry Clin Neurosci 2:429–431, 1990

Goldney RD, Spence ND: Safety of the combination of lithium and neuroleptic drugs. Am J Psychiatry 143:882–884, 1986

Gore CP, Egan GP, Walton D: The place of reserpine in the treatment of the chronic psychotic patient. Am J Psychiatry 114:333–337, 1957

Greendyke RM, Kanter DR: Plasma propranolol levels and their effect on plasma thioridazine and haloperidol concentrations. J Clin Psychopharmacol 7:178–182, 1987

Growe GA, Crayton JW, Klass DB, et al: Lithium in chronic schizophrenia. Am J Psychiatry 136:454–455, 1979

Hakola HPA, Laulumaa VA: Carbamazepine in treatment of violent schizophrenics (letter). Lancet 1:1358, 1982

Heh CWC, Sramek J, Herrera J, et al: Exacerbation of psychosis after discontinuation of carbamazepine treatment. Am J Psychiatry 145:878–879, 1988

Henry DA, Lawson DH, Reavey P, et al: Hyponatremia during carbamazepine treatment. BMJ 1:83–84, 1977

Herrera JM, Sramek JJ, Costa JF: Efficacy of adjunctive carbamazepine in the treatment chronic schizophrenia. Drug Intelligence and Clinical Pharmacy 21:355–358, 1987

Hogarty GE: Prevention of relapse in chronic schizophrenic patients. J Clin Psychiatry 54 (suppl 3):18–23, 1993

Hwang MY, Martin AM, Lindenmayer JP, et al: Treatment of schizophrenia with obsessive-compulsive features with serotonin reuptake inhibitors (letter). Am J Psychiatry 150:1127, 1993

Jann MW, Ereshefsky L, Saklad SR, et al: Effects of carbamazepine on plasma haloperidol levels. J Clin Psychopharmacol 5:106–109, 1985

Jann MW, Fidone GS, Hernandez JM, et al: Clinical implications of increased antipsychotic plasma concentrations upon anticonvulsant cessation. Psychiatry Res 28:153–159, 1989

Javitt DC, Zukin SR: Recent advances in the phencyclidine model of schizophrenia. Am J Psychiatry 148:1301–1308, 1991

Johnson RM, Seibyl J, Erdos J, et al: Mazindol augmentation of neuroleptics in cocaine abusers (NR182), in New Research Program and Abstracts: American Psychiatric Association 145th Annual Meeting, Washington, DC, May 2–7, 1992, p 92

Jones RW, Wesnes KA, Kirby J: Effects of NMDA modulation in scopolamine dementia. Ann N Y Acad Sci 640:241–244, 1991

Jose CJ, Perez-Cruet J: Incidence and morbidity of self-induced water intoxication in state mental hospital patients. Am J Psychiatry 136:221–222, 1979

Kahn D, Stevenson E, Douglas CJ: Effect of sodium valproate in three patients with organic brain syndromes. Am J Psychiatry 145:1010–1011, 1988

Kahn EM, Schulz SC, Perel JM, et al: Change in haloperidol level due to carbamazepine—a complicating factor in combined medication for schizophrenia. J Clin Psychopharmacol 10:54–57, 1990

Kane JM: The current status of neuroleptic therapy. J Clin Psychiatry 50:322–328, 1989

Karper LP, Seibyl JP, Krystal JH: Valproate management of psychosis in a patient with carbamazepine-induced hyponatremia. J Clin Psychopharmacol 12:137–139, 1992

Kidron R, Averbuch I, Klein E, et al: Carbamazepine-induced reduction of blood levels of haloperidol in chronic schizophrenia. Biol Psychiatry 20:219–222, 1985

Klein E, Bental E, Lerer B, et al: Carbamazepine and haloperidol vs placebo and haloperidol in excited psychoses. Arch Gen Psychiatry 41:165–170, 1984

Ko GN, Korpi ER, Freed WJ, et al: Effect of valproic acid on behavior and plasma amino acid concentrations in chronic schizophrenic patients. Biol Psychiatry 20:209–215, 1985

Kosten TA, Kosten TR: Pharmacological blocking agents for treating substance abuse. J Nerv Ment Dis 179:583–592, 1991

Kramer MS, Vogel WH, DiJohnson C, et al: Antidepressants in 'depressed' schizophrenic inpatients: a controlled trial. Arch Gen Psychiatry 46:922–928, 1989

Krystal JH, Karper LP, Seibyl JP, et al: Subanesthetic effects of the noncompetitive NMDA antagonist, ketamine, in humans: psychotomimetic, perceptual, cognitive, and neuroendocrine responses. Arch Gen Psychiatry 51:199–214, 1994

Lerner Y, Mintzer Y, Schestatzky M: Lithium combined with haloperidol in schizophrenic patients. Br J Psychiatry 153:359–362, 1988

Lindenmayer JP, Vakharia M, Kanofsky D: Fluoxetine in chronic schizophrenia (letter). J Clin Psychopharmacol 10:76, 1990

Lindstrom LH, Persson E: Propranolol in chronic schizophrenia: a controlled study in neuroleptic-treated patients. Br J Psychiatry 137:126–130, 1980

Linnoila M, Viukari M, Hietala O: Effect of sodium valproate on tardive dyskinesia. Br J Psychiatry 129:114–119, 1976

Lipinski JF Jr, Zubenko GS, Cohen BM, et al: Propranolol in the treatment of neuroleptic-induced akathisia. Am J Psychiatry 141:412–415, 1984

Lipinski JF Jr, Keck PE Jr, McElroy SL: Beta-adrenergic antagonists in psychosis: is improvement due to treatment of neuroleptic-induced akathisia? J Clin Psychopharmacol 8:409–416, 1988

Litman RE, Hong WW, Gutierrez R, et al: Idazoxan augmentation of neuroleptic therapy: antagonist strategies in the pharmacotherapy of schizophrenia (NR399), in New Research Program and Abstracts: American Psychiatric Association 145th Annual Meeting, Washington, DC, May 2–7, 1992, p 146

Luchins DJ: Carbamazepine for the violent psychiatric patient (letter). Lancet 1:766, 1983

Macklin EA, Simon A, Crook GH: Psychotic reactions in problem drinkers treated with disulfiram (Antabuse). AMA Archives of Neurology and Psychiatry 69:415–426, 1953

McElroy SL, Keck PE Jr, Pope HG Jr, et al: Valproate in psychiatric disorders: literature review and clinical guidelines. J Clin Psychiatry 50 (suppl 3):23–29, 1989

Miller FA, Rampling D: Adverse effects of combined propranolol and chlorpromazine therapy. Am J Psychiatry 139:1198–1199, 1982

Myers DH, Campbell PL, Cocks NM, et al: A trial of propranolol in chronic schizophrenia. Br J Psychiatry 139:118–121, 1981

Nagao T, Ohshimo T, Mitsunobu K, et al: Cerebrospinal fluid monoamine metabolites and cyclic nucleotides in chronic schizophrenic patients with tardive dyskinesia or drug-induced tremor. Biol Psychiatry 14:509–523, 1979

Neppe VM: Carbamazepine as adjunctive treatment in nonepileptic chronic inpatients with EEG temporal lobe abnormalities. J Clin Psychiatry 44:326–331, 1983

Newcomer JW, Faustman WO, Zipursky RB, et al: Zacopride in schizophrenia: a single-blind serotonin type 3 antagonist trial. Arch Gen Psychiatry 49:751–752, 1992

Nussenzveig IZ, Javitt DC, Silipo GS, et al: High-dose of glycine in the treatment of schizophrenia (NR98), in New Research Program and Abstracts: American Psychiatric Association 145th Annual Meeting, Washington, DC, May 2–7, 1992, p 71

Okuma T, Yamashita I, Takahashi R, et al: A double-blind study of adjunctive carbamazepine versus placebo on excited states of schizophrenia and schizoaffective disorders. Acta Psychiatr Scand 80:250–259, 1989

O'Malley SS, Jaffe AJ, Chang G, et al: Naltrexone and coping skills therapy for alcohol dependence: a controlled study. Arch Gen Psychiatry 49:881–887, 1992

Peet M, Bethell MS, Coates A, et al: Propranolol in schizophrenia, I: comparison of propranolol, chlorpromazine and placebo. Br J Psychiatry 139:105–111, 1981a

Peet M, Middlemiss DN, Yates RA: Propranolol in schizophrenia, II: clinical and biochemical aspects of combining propranolol with chlorpromazine. Br J Psychiatry 139:112–117, 1981b

Perenyi A, Goswami U, Frecska E, et al: L-Deprenyl in treating negative symptoms of schizophrenia (letter). Psychiatry Res 42:189–191, 1992

Pickar D, Wolkowitz OM, Doran AR, et al: Clinical and biochemical effects of verapamil administration to schizophrenic patients. Arch Gen Psychiatry 44:113–118, 1987

Pickar D, Owen RR, Litman RE: New developments in the pharmacotherapy of schizophrenia, in American Psychiatric Press Review of Psychiatry, Vol 10. Edited by Tasman A, Goldfinger SM. Washington, DC, American Psychiatric Press, 1991, pp 98–115

Pope HG Jr, McElroy SL, Satlin A, et al: Head injury, bipolar disorder, and response to valproate. Compr Psychiatry 29:34–38, 1988

Pope HG Jr, McElroy SL, Keck PE Jr, et al: Valproate in the treatment of acute mania: a placebo-controlled study. Arch Gen Psychiatry 48:62–68, 1991

Post RM, Weiss SR, Pert A: Differential effects of carbamazepine and lithium on sensitization and kindling. Prog Neuropsychopharmacol Biol Psychiatry 8:425–434, 1984

Post RM, Trimble MR, Pippenger CE: Clinical Use of Anticonvulsants in Psychiatric Disorders. New York, Demos Publications, 1989

Prakash R, Kelwala S, Ban TA: Neurotoxicity in patients with schizophrenia during lithium therapy. Compr Psychiatry 23:271-273, 1982a

Prakash R, Kelwala S, Ban TA: Neurotoxicity with combined administration of lithium and a neuroleptic. Compr Psychiatry 23:567–571, 1982b

Prien RF, Caffey EM, Klett CJ: A comparison of lithium carbonate and chlorpromazine in the treatment of excited schizo-affectives. Arch Gen Psychiatry 27:182–189, 1972

Pugh CR, Steinert J, Priest RG: Propranolol in schizophrenia: a double-blind, placebo-controlled trial of propranolol as an adjunct to neuroleptic medication. Br J Psychiatry 143:151–155, 1983

Ratey JJ, Sorgi P, O'Driscoll GA, et al: Nadolol to treat aggression and psychiatric symptomatology in chronic psychiatric inpatients: a double-blind, placebo-controlled study. J Clin Psychiatry 53:41–46, 1992

Reiter S, Adler L, Angrist B, et al: Effects of verapamil on tardive dyskinesia and psychosis in schizophrenic patients. J Clin Psychiatry 50:26–27, 1989

Rifkin A, Quitkin F, Klein DF: Organic brain syndrome during lithium carbonate treatment. Compr Psychiatry 14:251–254, 1973

Ross JL, MacKenzie TB, Hanson DR, et al: Diltiazem for tardive dyskinesia (letter). Lancet 1:268, 1987

Rosse RB, Schwartz BL, Davis RE, et al: An NMDA intervention strategy in schizophrenia with "low-dose" milacemide. Clin Neuropharmacol 14:268–272, 1991

Salzman C, Green AI, Rodriguez-Villa F, et al: Benzodiazepines combined with neuroleptics for management of severe disruptive behavior. Psychosomatics 27 (suppl):17–21, 1986

Scher M, Neppe V: Carbamazepine adjunct for nonresponsive psychosis with prior hallucinogenic abuse. J Nerv Ment Dis 177:755–757, 1989

Schou M: Lithium prophylaxis: myths and realities. Am J Psychiatry 146:573–576, 1989

Schulz SC, Kahn EM, Baker RW, et al: Lithium and carbamazepine augmentation in treatment-refractory schizophrenia, in The Neuroleptic-Nonresponsive Patient: Characterization and Treatment. Edited by Angrist B, Schulz SC. Washington, DC, American Psychiatric Press, 1990, pp 109–136

Seibyl JP, Brenner L, Krystal JH, et al: Mazindol and cocaine addiction in schizophrenia. Biol Psychiatry 31:1179–1181, 1992a

Seibyl J, Erdos J, Karper LP, et al: Long-term mazindol augmentation of neuroleptic in negative schizophrenia (Abstract 95.4). Society for Neuroscience Abstracts 18:202, 1992b

Sheard MH, Marini JL, Bridges CI, et al: The effect of lithium in impulsive aggressive behavior in man. Am J Psychiatry 133:1409–1413, 1976

Shopsin B, Kim SS, Gershon S: A controlled study of lithium vs. chlorpromazine in acute schizophrenics. Br J Psychiatry 119:435–440, 1971

Silver H, Nassar A: Fluvoxamine improves negative symptoms in treated chronic schizophrenia: an add-on double-blind, placebo-controlled study. Biol Psychiatry 31:698–704, 1992

Silver H, Blacker M, Weller MPI, et al: The treatment of chronic schizophrenia with cyproheptadine. Biol Psychiatry 25:502–504, 1989

Silver H, Blacker M, Weller MPI, et al: Treatment of chronic schizophrenia with cyproheptadine: a double-blind placebo-controlled study. Biol Psychiatry 30:523–525, 1991

Silver JM, Hales RE, Yudofsky SC: Psychiatric consultation to neurology, in American Psychiatric Press Review of Psychiatry, Vol 9. Edited by Tasman A, Goldfinger SM, Kaufmann C. Washington, DC, American Psychiatric Press, 1990, pp 433–465

Siris SG: Pharmacological treatment of depression in schizophrenia, in Depression in Schizophrenia. Edited by DeLisi LE. Washington, DC, American Psychiatric Press, 1990, pp 141–162

Siris SG, Morgan V, Fagerstrom R, et al: Adjunctive imipramine in the treatment of post-psychotic depression: a controlled trial. Arch Gen Psychiatry 44:533–539, 1987

Siris SG, Bermanzohn PC, Gonzalez A, et al: The use of antidepressants for negative symptoms in a subset of schizophrenic patients. Psychopharmacol Bull 27:331–335, 1991

Skuster DZ, Digre KB, Corbett JJ: Neurological conditions presenting as psychiatric disorders. Psychiatr Clin North Am 15:311–333, 1992

Slater E, Beard AW: The schizophrenia-like psychoses of epilepsy. Br J Psychiatry 109:95–150, 1963

Small JG, Kellams JJ, Milstein V, et al: A placebo-controlled study of lithium combined with neuroleptics in chronic schizophrenic patients. Am J Psychiatry 132:1315–1317, 1975

Sorgi PJ, Ratey JJ, Polakoff S: β-Adrenergic blockers for the control of aggressive behaviors in patients with chronic schizophrenia. Am J Psychiatry 143:775–776, 1986

Spring G, Frankel M: New data on lithium and haloperidol incompatibility. Am J Psychiatry 138:818–821, 1981

Sramek J, Herrera J, Costa J, et al: A carbamazepine trial in chronic, treatment-refractory schizophrenia. Am J Psychiatry 145:748–750, 1988

Stedman TJ, Whiteford HA, Eyles D, et al: Effects of nifedipine on psychosis and tardive dyskinesia in schizophrenic patients. J Clin Psychopharmacol 11:43–47, 1991

Stevens JR, Livermore A: Kindling of the mesolimbic dopamine system: animal model of psychosis. Neurology 28:36–46, 1978

Suddath RL, Straw GM, Freed WJ, et al: A clinical trial of nifedipine in schizophrenia and tardive dyskinesia. Pharmacol Biochem Behav 39:743–745, 1991

Tamminga CA, Schaffer MH: Treatment of schizophrenia with ergot derivatives. Psychopharmacology 66:239–242, 1979

Task Force on Tardive Dyskinesia: Tardive Dyskinesia: A Task Force Report of the American Psychiatric Association. Washington, DC, American Psychiatric Association, 1992, pp 180–182

Tupin JP, Smith DB, Clanon TL, et al: The long-term use of lithium in aggressive prisoners. Compr Psychiatry 14:311–317, 1973

Uhde TW, Post RM: Effects of carbamazepine on serum electrolytes: clinical and theoretical implications. J Clin Psychopharmacol 3:103–106, 1983

VanValkenburg C, Kluznik J, Merrill R, et al: Therapeutic levels of valproate for psychosis. Psychopharmacol Bull 26:254–255, 1990

Vieweg V, Glick JL, Herring S, et al: Absence of carbamazepine-induced hyponatremia among patients also given lithium. Am J Psychiatry 144:943–947, 1987

Wassef A, Watson DJ, Morrison P, et al: Neuroleptic-valproic acid combination in treatment of psychotic symptoms: a three-case report. J Clin Psychopharmacol 9:45–48, 1989

Waxman SG, Geschwind N: Hypergraphia in temporal lobe epilepsy. Neurology 24:629–636, 1974

Waxman SG, Geschwind N: The interictal behavior syndrome of temporal lobe epilepsy. Arch Gen Psychiatry 32:1580–1586, 1975

Waziri R: Glycine therapy of schizophrenia. Biol Psychiatry 23:210–211, 1988

Weiner N: Drugs that inhibit adrenergic nerves and block adrenergic receptors, in The Pharmacological Basis of Therapeutics, 7th Edition. Edited by Gilman AG, Goodman LS, Rall TW, et al. New York, Macmillan, 1985, pp 207–210

Wilson WH, Ban TA, Guy W: Pharmacotherapy of chronic hospitalized schizophrenics: prescription practices. Neuropsychobiology 14:75–82, 1985

Wolf MA, Diener JM, Lajeunesse C, et al: Low-dose bromocriptine in neuroleptic-resistant schizophrenia: a pilot study. Biol Psychiatry 31:1166–1168, 1992

Wolkowitz OM, Pickar D: Benzodiazepines in the treatment of schizophrenia: a review and reappraisal. Am J Psychiatry 148:714–726, 1991

Wolkowitz OM, Turetsky N, Reus VI, et al: Benzodiazepine augmentation of neuroleptics in treatment-resistant schizophrenia. Psychopharmacol Bull 28:291–295, 1992

Yorkston NJ, Zaki SA, Weller MP, et al: DL-propranolol and chlorpromazine following admission for schizophrenia: a controlled comparison. Acta Psychiatr Scand 63:13–27, 1981

Yudofsky S, Williams D, Gorman J: Propranolol in the treatment of rage and violent behavior in patients with chronic brain syndromes. Am J Psychiatry 138:218–220, 1981

Zemlen FP, Hirschowitz J, Sautter FJ, et al: Impact of lithium therapy on core psychotic symptoms of schizophrenia. Br J Psychiatry 144:64–69, 1984

Ziedonis D, Richardson T, Lee E, et al: Adjunctive desipramine in the treatment of cocaine abusing schizophrenics. Psychopharmacol Bull 28:309–314, 1992

CHAPTER 7

Noradrenergic Systems: A Target for Augmenting Pharmacotherapy

Robert E. Litman, M.D.
David Pickar, M.D.

One explanation for treatment resistance and partial response to the traditional dopamine-blocking neuroleptic drugs may be that neurotransmitter systems other than dopamine are disturbed in schizophrenia. If so, pharmacotherapy that targets other neurotransmitter systems may ultimately be more beneficial for patients with schizophrenia. In this chapter, we review the evidence that suggests that the noradrenergic system (i.e., the neurotransmitter norepinephrine [NE; Figure 7–1], its neurons, and its receptors in the brain) is an important target for pharmacotherapy in schizophrenia. We first provide an overview of the scientific evidence for disturbed noradrenergic function in schizophrenia. Next, we discuss the clinical use of noradrenergic agents in the pharmacotherapy of patients with schizophrenia, including specific indications, clinical efficacy, and side effects. Finally, we present a new rationale for targeting noradrenergic systems in the pharmacotherapy of schizophrenia, based on the unique pharmacology and biochemical effects of the atypical neuroleptic clozapine.

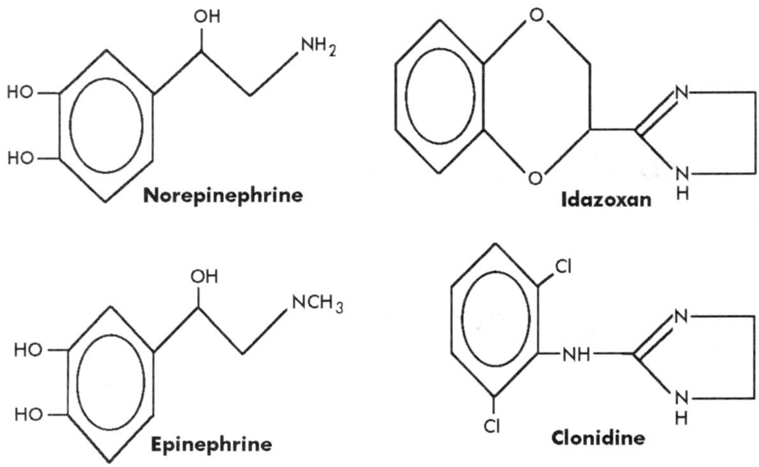

Figure 7–1. Chemical structure of the selective α_2 antagonist idazoxan compared with other compounds that act at adrenergic receptor sites.

Evidence for a Disturbance in Noradrenergic Neurotransmission in Schizophrenia

The dopamine hypothesis of schizophrenia posits that schizophrenic symptoms are caused by an overactivity of dopamine systems in the brain; however, this hypothesis is limited by the relative paucity of evidence for increased dopaminergic activity in schizophrenia. In contrast, several lines of evidence indicate that noradrenergic activity is altered in patients with schizophrenia (van Kammen and Kelley 1991). For example, postmortem studies have found increases in NE and its metabolites in the brains of patients with schizophrenia; these increases are localized to brain regions that are hypothesized to be involved in the pathophysiology of schizophrenia, including the nucleus accumbens, certain limbic nuclei, the basal ganglia, and the midbrain (Bird et al. 1979; Crow et al. 1979; Farley et al. 1978; Kleinman et al. 1979). Increases in NE and its metabolites have also been reported in the cerebrospinal fluid (CSF) and plasma of patients with schizophrenia (Albus et al. 1982; Breier et al. 1990; Castellani et al. 1982; Gomes et al. 1980; Lake et al. 1980); although some of these increases may be attributable to the effects of neuroleptic medication (Bagdy et al. 1985; Gattaz et al. 1983), increases have also been reported in patients who have not taken neuroleptic drugs for a long time and in neuroleptic-naive patients (Kemali et al. 1990; Sternberg et al. 1981).

Moreover, changes in NE and its metabolites have been found to correlate with psychopathology in schizophrenia. For example, increases in NE in postmortem brain tissue, plasma, and CSF are found primarily in patients with the paranoid subtype of schizophrenia or with high levels of paranoid symptoms (Albus et al. 1982; Farley et al. 1978; Gattaz et al. 1983; Kemali et al. 1990; Kleinman et al. 1979). High plasma and CSF levels of NE and its metabolite, 3-methoxy-4-hydroxyphenylglycol (MHPG), have been found to be significantly correlated with the clinical characteristics of patients with schizophrenia, including the severity of psychosis (Ko et al. 1988), relapse of psychosis (van Kammen et al. 1989, 1990), positive and negative symptom subtypes (Breier et al. 1990; Maas et al. 1993; Pickar et al. 1990; van Kammen et al. 1990), and favorable response to neuroleptic treatment (Bowers et al. 1987; Chang et al. 1990). In addition, decreases in noradrenergic indices during antipsychotic treatment with D_2 antagonist drugs (haloperidol and pimozide) have been found to parallel clinical improvement (Chang et al. 1990; Kaneko et al. 1992; Sternberg et al. 1981). In light of observations that noradrenergic indices may vary greatly with changes in clinical state, several groups have suggested that noradrenergic function is best understood as a state-dependent variable in patients with schizophrenia. van Kammen and colleagues (1989, 1990) have proposed that acute elevations in NE may constitute a prodrome for relapse of psychosis in certain patients with schizophrenia.

Impaired noradrenergic receptor function has also been investigated in patients with schizophrenia. The findings of blunted physiological response to pharmacological challenge with the α_2-receptor agonist clonidine (e.g., blunted decrease in plasma MHPG or blunted release of growth hormone) in several studies, as well as hypofunction of platelet α_2 receptors, suggest that α_2 receptors in patients with schizophrenia are functionally subsensitive (Kafka and van Kammen 1983; Sternberg et al. 1982). Subsensitivity of α_2 receptors might account for state-dependent increases in levels of NE observed in patients with schizophrenia because normally functioning presynaptic α_2 receptors inhibit NE release from the presynaptic neuron. However, abnormalities in response to pharmacological challenge with either clonidine or the α_2-receptor antagonist yohimbine are not found consistently in all patients or in all studies; indeed, evidence for α_2-receptor supersensitivity has been reported (Glazer et al. 1987; van Kammen and Kelley 1991). Similarly, results of studies of platelet α_2-receptor function have been inconsistent and difficult to interpret because of various methodological issues and confounds (Wirz-Justice 1988). Thus, it is unknown whether α_2-adrenergic-receptor function is impaired in schizophrenia. Future research that might clarify the dynamics of α_2-receptor function in schizophrenia will probably involve the investigation of postreceptor, intracellular mechanisms (e.g., α_2-receptor-linked inhibitory G proteins) that mediate signal transduction processes resulting from the binding of NE to α_2 receptors (Manji 1992).

Use of Noradrenergic Agents in the Pharmacotherapy of Schizophrenia

In this section, we review the therapeutic use of pharmacological agents that exert their effects on noradrenergic systems. We discuss pharmacologically nonspecific agents that nonetheless have prominent noradrenergic effects (e.g., neuroleptics and antidepressants) and agents that are relatively specific for noradrenergic receptors (e.g., clonidine and propranolol).

Neuroleptics

Note that a large number of commonly used neuroleptics affect noradrenergic neurotransmission as a result of their ability to block noradrenergic receptors, particularly α_1 receptors. Although these properties are believed to account for the autonomic side effects of these drugs (e.g., hypotension), some investigators have proposed that the neuroleptics' ability to block α_1 receptors may be related to their antipsychotic properties, based on correlations between clinical doses of neuroleptics and their effects on NE-mediated neuronal activity (Cohen and Lipinski 1986). Although a drug treatment trial of the potent α_1-blocker prazosin as a sole pharmacological treatment in patients with schizophrenia did not reduce psychotic symptoms (Hommer et al. 1984), it has been suggested that combining potent α_1 blockade with dopamine-receptor antagonism in pharmacological therapy may improve treatment efficacy. This combination has been proposed as a possible mechanism for clozapine's superior efficacy and lack of extrapyramidal side effects (Baldessarini et al. 1992; Deutch et al. 1991; Lane et al. 1988).

Tricyclic Antidepressants

The tricyclic antidepressants (TCAs) have been hypothesized to exert antidepressant effects, at least in part, on the basis of their abilities to block NE reuptake and to downregulate α- and β-adrenergic receptors (Heninger and Charney 1987). The use of TCAs in the pharmacotherapy of schizophrenia arises from the recognition that at least 25% of patients with schizophrenia may develop secondary ("postpsychotic") depression during the course of their illness (Siris et al. 1994) and that in a significant proportion of these patients, suicide may result (Roy 1986). Several well-controlled studies suggest that patients with schizophrenia and secondary depression who are otherwise stable may benefit from adjunctive use of TCAs with neuroleptic treatment. Note that these data suggest that antidepressants are effective only in a select, syndromally defined subset of patients who have schizophrenia and secondary depression and that antidepressant treatment primarily reduces symptoms of depression and related symptoms (Plasky 1991; Siris et al. 1994). Negative symptoms, which may overlap clinically with depression, are less likely to respond. However, at least one study suggests that adjunctive pharmacotherapy with TCAs may reduce negative symptoms (Siris et al. 1991; Wolkowitz 1993).

Core symptoms of psychosis do not respond to TCAs and, in fact, may be exacerbated by TCA treatment in unstable, acutely or subacutely ill patients or in patients not receiving concurrent neuroleptic treatment (Kramer et al. 1989); therefore, antidepressant treatment should be initiated only after psychotic symptoms have been well controlled on stable doses of antipsychotics. Once TCAs are started, sufficient time for treatment trial should be allowed because it may require more time to achieve an antidepressant effect in patients with schizophrenia compared with nonschizophrenic depressed subjects (Wolkowitz 1993). Cardiac and anticholinergic side effects should monitored, especially during the concomitant use of TCAs with low-potency antipsychotics and antiparkinsonian medications. Finally, because elevated plasma levels of both TCAs and neuroleptics may occur with concomitant use, plasma-level determinations are recommended during optimal adjunctive TCA treatment and with any changes in medication (Plasky 1991; Siris et al. 1988; Wolkowitz 1993).

Clonidine

Clonidine is a selective agonist of α-adrenergic receptors, particularly α_2 receptors. Stimulation of α_2 presynaptic receptors by clonidine results in inhibition of NE release. The hypothesis that the increases in NE levels observed in patients with schizophrenia are due to subsensitive α_2 receptors (as noted above) provides a rationale for the therapeutic use of a drug such as clonidine in patients with schizophrenia. Clonidine would inhibit noradrenergic function by enhancing α_2-receptor function (Sternberg et al. 1982). However, results of studies using clonidine to treat psychotic symptoms are, at best, mixed. Although data from the only controlled study of clonidine treatment suggested significant improvement in eight patients, other studies found no improvement or exacerbation of psychotic symptoms with clonidine. Positive response to clonidine occurred in patients with prior good response to neuroleptics or in patients with tardive dyskinesia, for which clonidine has been reported to be beneficial; patients who were resistant to neuroleptic treatment did not improve (Bond 1986; Donaldson et al. 1983; Meltzer 1986). Thus, the clinical indications for clonidine treatment in schizophrenia are unclear, especially given its hypotensive and sedative effects. It is interesting that one study found that clonidine treatment improved memory function in patients with schizophrenia, independent of its effects on psychosis (Fields et al. 1988). These findings may have implications for putative prefrontal cortical dysfunction in schizophrenia because clonidine has also been shown to improve memory function in nonhuman primates with prefrontal cortical lesions (Fields et al. 1988).

Propranolol

Propranolol is a β-adrenergic-receptor antagonist that has been used in the treatment of a variety of medical conditions, ranging from cardiovascular disease and vascular headache to hyperthyroidism. Initial uncontrolled reports of the use of high doses (0.5–4.5 g/day) of propranolol in small numbers of schizophrenia patients suggested that it might also have significant antipsychotic effects (Atsmon et al. 1971; Elizur et al. 1979; Yorkston et al. 1974). Although some controlled studies showed that propranolol had beneficial effects on psychotic symptoms (Yorkston et al. 1977), negative symptoms (Eccleston et al. 1985), and nonspecific symptoms of anxiety, irritability, or agitation (Lindstrom and Persson 1980), the majority of controlled studies showed minimal or no antipsychotic effects of this drug (Christison et al. 1991; Donaldson et al. 1983; Lader 1988). Several reviews note that the antipsychotic effects of propranolol occur primarily in patients who are also receiving neuroleptic treatment and that this may be due to propranolol's reported ability to increase plasma neuroleptic levels (Donaldson et al. 1983; Lader 1988; Peet 1981; Wolkowitz 1993). Another reason that propranolol may help patients is the ameliorative effects of the β-blockers on neuroleptic-induced akathisia (Lipinski et al. 1988). Thus, use of propranolol may be best reserved for the subgroup of patients whose resistance to neuroleptic treatment is due to severe akathisia. Propranolol also may be useful for treatment-resistant patients with coarse brain disease or high degrees of aggressivity (Donaldson et al. 1983; Wolkowitz 1993). In any case, indications for using propranolol in the pharmacotherapy of schizophrenia are limited, especially because of its potential for serious cardiovascular side effects (e.g., hypotension and bradycardia).

Clozapine and Norepinephrine: A New Rationale for Targeting Noradrenergic Systems in the Pharmacotherapy of Schizophrenia

In what may prove to be a landmark study, John Kane and colleagues (1988) convincingly demonstrated that the atypical neuroleptic clozapine had significantly greater antipsychotic efficacy than typical neuroleptic drugs in the pharmacotherapy of treatment-refractory patients with schizophrenia. Clozapine's superior efficacy is thought to be based, at least in part, on its ability to influence the function of a broad spectrum of neurotransmitter systems. In addition to its antagonism of dopamine receptors, clozapine is a potent antagonist of adrenergic, muscarinic, histaminic, and serotonergic receptors. Although it has been suggested that clozapine's unique ratio of serotonin-to-dopamine receptor binding is a central component of its antipsychotic mechanism (Meltzer 1989), clozapine's ability to enhance noradrenergic neurotransmission may be an additional distinguishing biochemical feature. In a double-blind, pharmacological crossover study that compared clozapine with the typical neuroleptic fluphenazine in 21 patients with schizophrenia, we found that clozapine significantly elevated plasma levels of NE and normetanephrine (a metabolite of NE) (Pickar et al. 1992); in addition, urinary noradrenergic indices suggested that clozapine treatment increased noradrenergic release and turnover (W. Z. Potter, personal communication, May 1992). Several laboratories have independently confirmed these effects of clozapine on plasma levels of NE in patients with schizophrenia (Breier et al. 1994; Davidson et al. 1993; Green et al. 1993); one study reported that clozapine-induced increased plasma levels of NE correlated with positive response to clozapine treatment (Breier et al. 1994).

It is not clear how clozapine acts to increase plasma levels of NE. One possible explanation is clozapine's antagonism of α_2-adrenergic receptors, which is more potent than that of typical neuroleptic agents (Richelson and Nelson 1984). This antagonism would diminish negative feedback inhibition of the presynaptic α_2 receptor and result in increased NE release. Other more recent evidence suggests that clozapine may block the reuptake of released NE, which would also result in increased plasma levels of NE (Breier et al. 1994). Whatever the mechanism underlying the increase in NE, we hypothesized that this effect of clozapine might be relevant to its antipsychotic mechanism; this, in turn, led to our interest in using other agents in the pharmacotherapy of patients with schizophrenia, which, like clozapine, would enhance noradrenergic neurotransmission.

Use of Idazoxan to Augment Treatment Response to Typical Neuroleptics in Patients With Schizophrenia

We hypothesized that a pharmacotherapeutic strategy that enhanced noradrenergic neurotransmission would reduce symptoms beyond that observed for typical neuroleptic treatment. Because we postulated that one mechanism for clozapine's noradrenergic effects might be antagonism of presynaptic α_2 receptors, we decided to use idazoxan, an experimental α_2-adrenergic-receptor antagonist (Figure 7–1), as a pharmacological treatment in patients with schizophrenia who were already stabilized on typical neuroleptics.

Idazoxan, an imidazoline compound, is a highly potent, highly selective antagonist of α_2-adrenergic receptors, with significantly higher affinity for α_2 receptors compared with other monoaminergic receptors (e.g., α_1, serotonin, and dopamine) (Doxey et al. 1984; Nicholson and Pascoe 1991). Note that, as an imidazoline derivative, idazoxan also binds nonadrenergic imidazoline receptor sites in the brain (Michel et al. 1989); however, the emotional and behavioral effects mediated by imidazoline-sensitive receptor sites are still unclear (Nicholson and Pascoe 1991). Idazoxan has been used safely in healthy volunteers as well as in patients with bipolar depression (Nicholson and Pascoe 1991; Osman et al. 1989). In a pilot study of six patients with treatment-resistant schizophrenia, we found that the addition of idazoxan to stable typical neuroleptic treatment significantly reduced psychiatric symptoms, especially negative symptoms, compared with typical neuroleptic treatment alone (Litman et al. 1993).

We continued to add idazoxan to stable neuroleptic treatment under double-blind, placebo-controlled conditions in 16 (5 female, 11 male) hospitalized patients who met DSM-III-R (American Psychiatric Association 1987) criteria and Research Diagnostic Criteria (Spitzer et al. 1978) for schizophrenia or schizoaffective disorder and who were judged to be resistant to treatment with typical neuroleptics (Litman et al. 1993; Pickar et al. 1992). For approximately 8 weeks, patients were treated with fluphenazine hydrochloride, adjusting the dosage to a level at which patients were judged to be clinically stable. Benztropine mesylate was also administered as needed for extrapyramidal side effects. Patients were maintained on stable doses of fluphenazine hydrochloride and benztropine for at least 2 weeks before the addition of idazoxan; doses of both fluphenazine hydrochloride and benztropine mesylate achieved during the stabilization period remained unchanged throughout the entire study.

Idazoxan was added at an initial dose of 20 mg bid and increased over 2 weeks to a fixed study dose of 120 mg/day. Five patients had to be maintained on lower fixed doses (80–100 mg/day) because of mild side effects, such as insomnia, headache, and tremor. Patients were treated with idazoxan for at least 4 weeks. Idazoxan was then tapered by reductions of 20 mg/day over 2 weeks. Following discontinuation of idazoxan, we studied patients on fluphenazine alone for an additional 3–4 weeks. All medications were administered under double-blind, placebo-controlled conditions (Figure 7–2).

Psychiatrists blind to medication status rated patients weekly with the Bunney-Hamburg Global Rating Scales for psychosis,

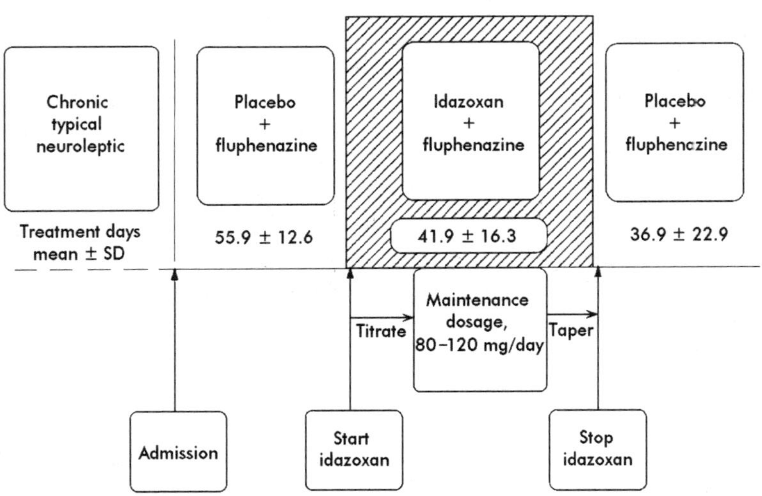

Figure 7–2. Study design, order, and length of medication administration in therapeutic trial of idazoxan plus fluphenazine in 16 patients with schizophrenia.

anxiety, mania, and depression (Bunney and Hamburg 1963); the modified 24-item Brief Psychiatric Rating Scale (BPRS; Overall and Gorham 1962); the Scale for the Assessment of Negative Symptoms (SANS; Andreasen 1981); the Abnormal Involuntary Movements Scale (AIMS; Guy 1976); and the Simpson Neurological Rating Scale (Simpson and Angus 1970) for drug side effects.

In the majority of patients, symptoms decreased significantly when idazoxan was added to stable fluphenazine treatment, and the symptoms returned to baseline levels after discontinuation of idazoxan. Idazoxan treatment resulted in significant reductions ($P < .01$) in global ratings of psychosis and in the BPRS total score compared with fluphenazine treatment alone before addition of idazoxan. Global psychosis ratings were also reduced significantly *after* discontinuation of idazoxan compared with ratings on fluphenazine ($P < .05$) (Figure 7–3 and Table 7–1). Both positive and negative symptom subtypes were significantly reduced by combination treatment of idazoxan plus fluphenazine compared with fluphenazine treatment alone before addition of idazoxan. Significant reductions in positive symptoms were reflected in decreases in the BPRS positive symptom subscale, as well as in decreases in individual positive symptoms, including unusual thought (item 13) ($P < .05$) and paranoia/suspiciousness (item 11) ($P > .01$); the latter symptom was also reduced compared with fluphenazine treatment after discontinuation of idazoxan ($P < .05$). Effects on negative symptoms were reflected in significant reductions ($P < .05$) in the BPRS negative symptom subscale, although idazoxan treatment did not affect negative symptom ratings on the SANS. No significant changes were found in Simpson Neurological Scale ratings of extrapyramidal symptoms or AIMS ratings of abnormal motor movements when idazoxan was added to chronic fluphenazine treatment (see Table 7–1).

These data suggest that the addition of idazoxan to stable neuroleptic treatment reduces symptoms in patients with schizophrenia who are resistant to neuroleptic treatment. Although the reduction is modest (10%–15% of BPRS total score), it is similar to that observed in studies of other nonneuroleptic drugs (e.g., antidepressants [Plasky 1991] and benzodiazepines [Wolkowitz et al. 1990]) used to augment response to neuroleptic therapy. In addition, several patients experienced greater reductions

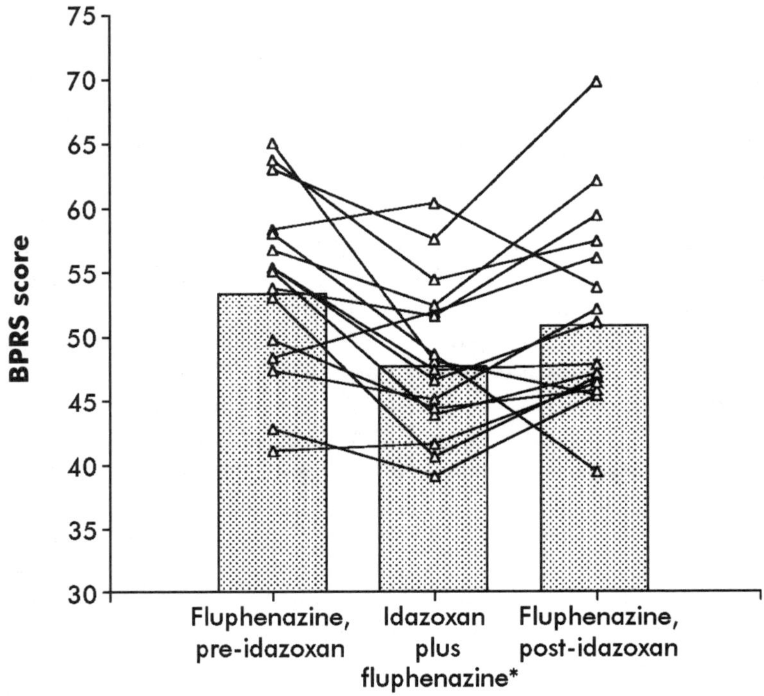

Figure 7–3. Changes in Brief Psychiatric Rating Scale (BPRS; Overall and Gorham 1962) total score during therapeutic trial of idazoxan plus fluphenazine in 16 patients with schizophrenia ($F = 6.15$, $P = .006$). *$P < .01$ in comparison to treatment with fluphenazine alone before the addition of idazoxan.

in symptoms, ranging from 20% to 30%. Both positive and negative symptoms were significantly reduced when idazoxan was added to fluphenazine. Moreover, the marked effect of this combination in reducing paranoia is noteworthy because other investigators have noted that noradrenergic abnormalities occur in patients with prominent paranoid symptoms (Bird et al. 1979; Crow et al. 1979; Farley et al. 1978; Kleinman et al. 1979). The reduction in symptoms with idazoxan was not due to reduction in global depression or mood symptoms or to the amelioration of extrapyramidal side effects. In addition, no increase or "rebound"

Table 7–1. Augmentation of response to typical neuroleptic using idazoxan: behavioral effects

	FLU, pre-IDX mean (SD)	FLU + IDX mean (SD)	FLU, post-IDX mean (SD)
Bunney-Hamburg Global Ratings			
Psychosis	5.4 (0.8)	4.8 (0.6)*,**	5.2 (0.8)
Depression	2.4 (0.9)	2.1 (0.7)	2.2 (0.8)
Anxiety	2.2 (1.0)	2.0 (0.7)	2.2 (0.8)
Mania	1.2 (0.4)	1.2 (0.5)	1.1 (0.3)
BPRS total	54.1 (7.0)	48.2 (6.0)*	51.5 (7.8)
Positive symptoms	10.1 (3.0)	8.7 (2.3)***	10.1 (2.7)
Negative symptoms	10.6 (2.5)	9.5 (1.7)***	10.0 (1.5)
Anxiety	2.9 (0.8)	2.3 (0.6)***	2.4 (0.8)
Guilt	2.4 (1.3)	1.7 (0.9)***	1.9 (1.4)
Paranoia/suspiciousness	3.7 (1.2)	2.9 (0.9)*,**	3.5 (1.2)
Unusual thought	2.7 (1.3)	2.2 (0.9)***	2.7 (1.4)
Simpson Neurological	12.6 (1.9)	12.4 (1.8)	12.4 (1.7)
AIMS	13.1 (1.9)	12.9 (1.6)	13.0 (1.6)
Plasma fluphenazine (ng/ml)	6.8 (5.6)	6.6 (4.6)	6.6 (4.4)

Note. AIMS = Abnormal Involuntary Movement Scale (Guy 1976), BPRS = Brief Psychiatric Rating Scale (Overall and Gorham 1962), FLU = fluphenazine treatment, IDX = idazoxan treatment, SD = standard deviation.
$^{*}P < .01$ compared with fluphenazine, pre-idazoxan. $^{**}P < .05$ compared with fluphenazine, post-idazoxan discontinuation. $^{***}P < .05$.

in psychosis was caused by withdrawal of idazoxan. Finally, repeated assay of fluphenazine in subgroups of patients did not show any effect of idazoxan on fluphenazine levels, indicating that the observed improvement was not related to a pharmacokinetic interaction of idazoxan with fluphenazine.

A serious limitation of this study is its fixed-order design (i.e., idazoxan was always administered with fluphenazine treatment); thus, the effects we attribute to idazoxan might be due, at least in part, to other factors such as the length of hospital stay. In order to test definitively the efficacy of combined idazoxan–typical neuroleptic treatment, a double-blind, controlled study in which parallel groups of patients are randomized to treatment with either idazoxan plus typical neuroleptic or placebo plus typical neuroleptic is warranted.

Nonetheless, these data support the notion that a pharmacotherapeutic strategy that enhances noradrenergic neurotransmission by increasing blockade of α_2-adrenergic receptors will augment neuroleptic response in patients with schizophrenia. These data also suggest that clozapine's effects on noradrenergic neurotransmission may be relevant to its mechanism of action. At present, it is not clear how increasing α_2 blockade with idazoxan reduces symptoms. Although the effect may be due to a direct modulation of noradrenergic function, increasing α_2 blockade may affect dopaminergic neurotransmission as a result of an interaction with dopamine systems. For example, α_2 blockade with idazoxan has been shown to increase firing in locus coeruleus (LC) noradrenergic neurons (Grenhoff and Svensson 1989, 1993); increased firing of LC neurons in the LC modulates firing of midbrain mesolimbic and mesocortical dopamine neurons (Grenhoff and Svensson 1989; Grenhoff et al. 1993). Alternatively, it is possible that dopamine and α_2-adrenergic receptors share the same inhibitory G protein (Manji 1992); thus, modulation of dopaminergic neurotransmission via α_2 blockade may also occur intraneuronally, during signal transduction. Whatever the mechanism, the behavioral effects we observed with idazoxan provide greater impetus for investigations into brain noradrenergic-dopaminergic interactions, which have long been suspected to be involved in the pathophysiology of schizophrenia (van Kammen and Kelley 1991).

Conclusion

One may conclude from our review that a rationale for targeting noradrenergic systems in the pharmacotherapy of patients with schizophrenia is still somewhat unclear. Although several lines of evidence suggest that some disturbance of noradrenergic function occurs in schizophrenia, the exact nature of this disturbance and its role in the pathophysiology of schizophrenia are unknown. Also, the fact that adrenergic agents generally lack antipsychotic efficacy does little to encourage this approach.

However, we believe that the pharmacology of clozapine may be the best reason to reconsider in a positive light the importance of NE, if not in the pathophysiology, then certainly in the pharmacotherapy of schizophrenia. Clozapine's effects on NE inspired us to test the hypothesis that increasing α_2 blockade would further improve treatment response in patients, and our data, although preliminary, suggest that this is indeed so. This experiment indicates the need for similar clinical investigations using agents selective for other neurotransmitter systems at which clozapine has potent effects (e.g., ritanserin for serotonergic receptors) in the pharmacotherapy of patients with schizophrenia. We believe that this type of investigation could further illuminate clozapine's antipsychotic mechanism and may ultimately lead to better pharmacotherapeutic approaches for patients with schizophrenia.

References

Albus M, Engel RR, Muller F, et al: Experimental stress situations and state of autonomic arousal in schizophrenic and depressed patients. International Pharmacopsychiatry 17:129–135, 1982

American Psychiatric Association: Diagnostic and Statistical Manual of Mental Disorders, 3rd Edition, Revised. Washington, DC, American Psychiatric Association, 1987

Andreasen NC: The Scale for the Assessment of Negative Symptoms (SANS). Iowa City, IA, University of Iowa, 1981

Atsmon A, Blum I, Wijsenbeek H, et al: The short-term effect of adrenergic-blocking agents in a small group of psychotic patients. Psychiatria, Neurologia, Neurochirugia 74:251–258, 1971

Bagdy G, Perenyi A, Frecska E, et al: Decrease in dopamine, its metabolites and noradrenaline in cerebrospinal fluid of schizophrenic patients after withdrawal of long-term neuroleptic treatment. Psychopharmacology (Berl) 85:62–64, 1985

Baldessarini RJ, Huston-Lyons A, Campbell A, et al: Do central antiadrenergic actions contribute to the atypical properties of clozapine? Br J Psychiatry 160 (suppl 17):12–16, 1992

Bird ED, Spokes EGS, Iversen LL: Increased dopamine concentration in limbic areas of brain from patients dying with schizophrenia. Brain 102:347–360, 1979

Bond WS: Psychiatric indications for clonidine: neuropharmacologic and clinical basis. J Clin Psychopharmacol 6:81–87, 1986

Bowers MB, Swigar ME, Hoffman FJ, et al: Early neuroleptic response: clinical profiles and plasma catecholamine metabolites. J Clin Psychopharmacol 7:83–86, 1987

Breier A, Wolkowitz OM, Roy A, et al: Plasma norepinephrine in chronic schizophrenia. Am J Psychiatry 147:1467–1469, 1990

Breier A, Buchanan RW, Waltrip RW, et al: Clozapine's effects on plasma norepinephrine: relationship to clinical efficacy. Neuropsychopharmacology 10:1–7, 1994

Bunney WE, Hamburg DA: Methods for reliable longitudinal observation of behavior. Arch Gen Psychiatry 9:280–294, 1963

Castellani S, Ziegler MG, van Kammen DP, et al: Plasma norepinephrine and dopamine β hydroxylase activity in schizophrenia. Arch Gen Psychiatry 39:1145–1149, 1982

Chang WH, Chen TY, Lin SK, et al: Plasma catecholamine metabolites in schizophrenics: evidence for the two-subtype concept. Biol Psychiatry 27:510–518, 1990

Christison GW, Kirch DG, Wyatt R: When symptoms persist: choosing among alternative somatic treatments for schizophrenia. Schizophr Bull 17:217–245, 1991

Cohen BM, Lipinski JF: In vivo potencies of antipsychotic drugs in blocking alpha 1 noradrenergic and dopamine D2 receptors: implications for drug mechanism of action. Life Sci 39:2571–2580, 1986

Crow TJ, Baker HF, Cross AJ, et al: Monoamine mechanisms in chronic schizophrenia: post-mortem neurochemical findings. Br J Psychiatry 134:249–256, 1979

Davidson M, Kahn RS, Hirschowitz J, et al: Treatment with clozapine and its effect on plasma homovanillic acid and norepinephrine concentrations in schizophrenia. Psychiatry Res 46:51–163, 1993

Deutch AY, Moghaddam B, Innis RB, et al: Mechanisms of action of atypical antipsychotic drugs: implications for novel therapeutic strategies for schizophrenia. Schizophr Res 4:121–156, 1991

Donaldson SR, Gelenberg AJ, Baldessarini RJ: The pharmacologic treatment of schizophrenia: a progress report. Schizophr Bull 9:504–527, 1983

Doxey JC, Lane AC, Roach AG, et al: Comparison of the α-adrenoreceptor antagonist profiles of idazoxan (RX 781094), yohimbine, rauwolscine, and corynanthine. Archives of Pharmacology 325:136–144, 1984

Eccleston D, Fairbairn AF, Hassanyeh F, et al: The effect of propranolol and thioridazine on positive and negative symptoms of schizophrenia. Br J Psychiatry 147:623–630, 1985

Elizur A, Segal Z, Yeret A, et al: Antipsychotic effect of propranolol on chronic schizophrenics: study of a gradual treatment regimen. Psychopharmacology (Berl) 60:189–194, 1979

Farley IJ, Price KS, McCullough E: Norepinephrine in chronic paranoid schizophrenia: above normal levels in limbic forebrain. Science 200:456–458, 1978

Fields EB, van Kammen DP, Peters JL, et al: Clonidine improves memory function in schizophrenia independently from change in psychosis: preliminary findings. Schizophr Res 1:417–423, 1988

Gattaz WF, Riederer P, Reynolds GP, et al: Dopamine and noradrenaline in the cerebrospinal fluid of schizophrenic patients. Psychiatry Res 8:243–250, 1983

Glazer WM, Charney DS, Heninger GR: Noradrenergic function in schizophrenia. Arch Gen Psychiatry 44:898–904, 1987

Gomes UCR, Shanely BC, Potgeiter L, et al: Noradrenergic overactivity in chronic schizophrenia: evidence based on cerebrospinal fluid noradrenaline and cyclic nucleotide concentrations. Br J Psychiatry 137:346–351, 1980

Green AI, Alam MY, Sobieraj JT, et al: Clozapine response and plasma catecholamines and their metabolites. Psychiatry Res 46:139–149, 1993

Grenhoff J, Svensson TH: Clonidine modulates dopamine cell firing in rat ventral tegmental area. Eur J Pharmacol 165:11–18, 1989

Grenhoff J, Svensson TH: Prazosin modulates the firing pattern of dopamine neurons in rat ventral tegmental area. Eur J Pharmacol 233:79–84, 1993

Grenhoff J, Nisell M, Ferre S, et al: Noradrenergic modulation of midbrain dopamine cell firing elicited by stimulation of the locus coeruleus in the rat. J Neural Transm 93:11–25, 1993

Guy W (ed): ECDEU Assessment Manual for Psychopharmacology, Revised (DHEW Publ No ADM 76-338). Rockville, MD, U.S. Department of Health, Education and Welfare, 1976

Heninger GR, Charney DS: Mechanism of action of antidepressant treatments: implications for the etiology and treatment of depressive disorders, in Psychopharmacology: The Third Generation of Progress. Edited by Meltzer HY. New York, Raven, 1987, pp 535–545

Hommer DW, Zahn TP, Pickar D, et al: Prazosin, a specific alpha$_1$-noradrenergic receptor antagonist, has no effect on symptoms but increases autonomic arousal in schizophrenic patients. Psychiatry Res 11:193–204, 1984

Kafka MS, van Kammen DP: Alpha-adrenergic receptor function in schizophrenia: receptor number, cyclic adenosine monophosphate production, adenylate cyclase activity and effects of drugs. Arch Gen Psychiatry 40:264–270, 1983

Kane J, Honigfeld G, Singer J, et al: Clozapine for the treatment-resistant schizophrenic: a double-blind comparison with chlorpromazine. Arch Gen Psychiatry 45:789–796, 1988

Kaneko M, Kyoichi H, Tomoyuki K, et al: Plasma free 3-methoxy-4-hydroxyphenylglycol in acute schizophrenics before and after treatment. Neuropsychobiology 25:126–129, 1992

Kemali D, Maj M, Galderisi S, et al: Factors associated with increased noradrenaline levels in schizophrenic patients. Prog Neuropsychopharmacol Biol Psychiatry 14:49–59, 1990

Kleinman JE, Bridge P, Karoum F, et al: Catecholamines and metabolites in the brains of psychotics and normals: postmortem studies, in Catecholamines: Basic and Clinical Frontiers, Vol 1. Edited by Usdin E, Kopin IJ, Barchas J. Elmsford, NY, Pergamon, 1979, pp 1845–1847

Ko GN, Jimerson DC, Richard JW, et al: Plasma 3-methoxy 4-hydroxyphenylglycol changes associated with clinical state and schizophrenic subtype. Arch Gen Psychiatry 45:842–846, 1988

Kramer MS, Vogel WH, DiJohnson C, et al: Antidepressants in 'depressed' schizophrenic inpatients. Arch Gen Psychiatry 46:922–928, 1989

Lader M: β adrenoreceptor antagonists in neuropsychiatry: an update. J Clin Psychiatry 49:213–223, 1988

Lake CR, Sternberg DE, van Kammen DP, et al: Schizophrenia: elevated cerebrospinal fluid norepinephrine. Science 207:331–333, 1980

Lane RF, Claha CD, Rivet JM: Selective inhibition of dopamine release following chronic administration of clozapine: involvement of α_1-noradrenergic receptors demonstrated by in vivo voltammetry. Brain Res 460:398–401, 1988

Lindstrom LH, Persson E: Propranolol in chronic schizophrenia: a controlled study in neuroleptic-treated patients. Br J Psychiatry 137:126–130, 1980

Lipinski JF, Keck PE, McElroy SL: β-adrenergic antagonists in psychosis: is improvement due to treatment of neuroleptic-induced akathisia? J Clin Psychopharmacol 8:409–416, 1988

Litman RE, Hong WW, Weissman EM, et al: Idazoxan, an α_2 antagonist, augments fluphenazine response in schizophrenic patients: a pilot study. J Clin Psychopharmacol 13:264–267, 1993

Maas JW, Contreras SA, Miller AL, et al: Studies of catecholamine metabolism in schizophrenia/psychosis, I. Neuropsychopharmacology 8:97–109, 1993

Manji HK: G-Proteins: implications for psychiatry. Am J Psychiatry 149:746–760, 1992

Meltzer HY: Novel approaches to the pharmacotherapy of schizophrenia. Drug Development Research 9:23–40, 1986

Meltzer HY: Clinical studies on the mechanism of action of clozapine: the dopamine-serotonin hypothesis of schizophrenia. Psychopharmacology (Berl) 99:S18–S27, 1989

Michel MC, Brodde OE, Schneppel B, et al: [^{3}H]Idazoxan and some other α_2-adrenergic drugs also bind with high affinity to nonadrenergic site. Mol Pharmacol 35:324–330, 1989

Nicholson AN, Pascoe PA: Presynaptic alpha2-adrenoceptor function and sleep in man: studies with clonidine and idazoxan. Neuropharmacology 30:367–372, 1991

Osman O, Rudorfer MV, Potter WZ: Idazoxan: a selective α_2-antagonist and effective sustained antidepressant in two bipolar depressed patients. Arch Gen Psychiatry 46:958–959, 1989

Overall JE, Gorham DE: The Brief Psychiatric Rating Scale. Psychol Rep 10:799–812, 1962

Peet M: Is propranolol antischizophrenic? Neuropharmacology 20:1303–1307, 1981

Pickar D, Breier A, Hsiao JK, et al: Cerebrospinal fluid and plasma monoamine metabolites and their relation to psychosis: implications for regional brain dysfunction in schizophrenia. Arch Gen Psychiatry 47:541–648, 1990

Pickar D, Owen RR, Litman RE, et al: Clinical and biologic response to clozapine in patients with schizophrenia: crossover comparison with fluphenazine. Arch Gen Psychiatry 49:345–353, 1992

Plasky P: Antidepressant usage in schizophrenia. Schizophr Bull 17:649–657, 1991

Richelson E, Nelson A: Antagonism by neuroleptics of neurotransmitter receptors of normal human brain in vitro. Eur J Pharmacol 103:197–204, 1984

Roy A: Depression, attempted suicide, and suicide in patients with chronic schizophrenia. Psychiatr Clin North Am 9:193–206, 1986

Simpson G, Angus JSW: A rating scale for extrapyramidal side effects. Acta Psychiatr Scand 212:S9–S11, 1970

Siris SG, Adan F, Lee A, et al: Patterns of plasma imipramine-desipramine concentrations in patients receiving concomitant fluphenazine decanoate. J Clin Psychiatry 49:64–65, 1988

Siris SG, Bermanzohn PC, Gonzalez A, et al: The use of antidepressants for negative symptoms in a subset of schizophrenic patients. Psychopharmacol Bull 27:331–335, 1991

Siris SG, Bermanzohn PC, Mason SE, et al: Maintenance imipramine therapy for secondary depression in schizophrenia: a controlled trial. Arch Gen Psychiatry 51:109–115, 1994

Spitzer RL, Endicott J, Robins E: Research Diagnostic Criteria: rationale and reliability. Arch Gen Psychiatry 35:773 782, 1978

Sternberg DE, van Kammen DP, Lake CR, et al: The effect of pimozide on CSF norepinephrine in schizophrenia. Am J Psychiatry 138:1045–1051, 1981

Sternberg DE, Charney DS, Heninger GR, et al: Impaired presynaptic regulation of norepinephrine in schizophrenia: effects of clonidine in schizophrenic patients and normal controls. Arch Gen Psychiatry 39:285–289, 1982

van Kammen DP, Kelley M: Dopamine and norepinephrine activity in schizophrenia: an integrative perspective. Schizophr Res 4:173–191, 1991

van Kammen DP, Peters J, van Kammen WB, et al: CSF norepinephrine in schizophrenia is elevated prior to relapse after haloperidol withdrawal. Biol Psychiatry 26:176–188, 1989

van Kammen DP, Peters J, van Kammen WB, et al: Norepinephrine in acute exacerbations of chronic schizophrenia. Arch Gen Psychiatry 47:161–168, 1990

Wirz-Justice A: Platelet research in psychiatry. Experentia 44:145–152, 1988

Wolkowitz O: Rational polypharmacy in schizophrenia. Annals of Clinical Psychiatry 5:79–90, 1993

Wolkowitz OM, Rapaport MH, Pickar D: Benzodiazepine augmentation of neuroleptics, in The Neuroleptic Nonresponsive Patient: Characterization and Treatment. Edited by Angrist B, Schulz SC. Washington, DC, American Psychiatric Press, 1990, pp 87–108

Yorkston NJ, Zaki SA, Mlik MKU, et al: Propranolol in the control of schizophrenic symptoms. BMJ 14:633–635, 1974

Yorkston NJ, Gruzeiler JH, Zaki SA, et al: Propranolol as an adjunct to the treatment of schizophrenia. Lancet 2:575–578, 1977

CHAPTER 8

Benzodiazepines

Owen M. Wolkowitz, M.D.

Although neuroleptics remain the major class of drugs used in the pharmacotherapy of schizophrenia, several problems limit their usefulness (Table 8–1). First, acute and chronic side effects (e.g., dystonias, akathisia, autonomic side effects, and tardive dyskinesia) may limit upward dosing and diminish compliance (Davis 1980; Pickar 1986). Second, neuroleptics may take weeks to months to reach peak efficacy (McDermott et al. 1991; Pickar 1988). Third, not all symptoms of schizophrenia respond equally well to neuroleptics. For example, "negative symptoms" such as emotional withdrawal, apathy, and blunted affect may respond differently from "positive symptoms" such as hallucinations, delusions, and thought disorder (Breier et al. 1987; Crow 1980). Finally, many patients with schizophrenia do not respond well to neuroleptic medication (Davis 1980). This latter issue takes on particular significance when it is considered that poorly controlled psychotic episodes may have long-term deleterious effects. Wyatt (1991), for example, suggested that unmitigated psychotic symptoms may be "biologically toxic" and have cumulative effects in much the same way that several cardiac ischemic attacks may lead to the development of chronic heart failure. The National Institute of Mental Health Longitudinal Study of Chronic Schizophrenia also suggested that treatments that reduce positive and negative symptoms acutely would be beneficial for the long-term course and outcome of schizophrenia (Breier et al. 1991a).

Table 8–1. Problems with neuroleptic treatment in schizophrenia

Problems with neuroleptics	**Desirable properties of adjunctive or alternative drugs**
Side effects	Benign side-effect profile
Time latency	Quick acting
Not all symptoms respond	Broad acting
Not all patients respond	Target nonresponders

Based on these problems with neuroleptics, the goals of alternative or adjunctive pharmacotherapy are to 1) lessen the incidence or severity of neuroleptic side effects, perhaps by allowing the use of lower neuroleptic doses; 2) hasten therapeutic response; 3) treat a broader range of schizophrenic symptoms; and 4) treat neuroleptic nonresponders (Table 8–1). Once conventional neuroleptic treatment has been optimized (Pickar 1986; Wolkowitz 1993; see also Chapter 5 in this volume) but response remains unsatisfactory, switching to an alternative antipsychotic (e.g., the atypical antipsychotic clozapine) or augmenting neuroleptic treatment with adjunctive drugs is a viable option. Some controversy exists about which approach to try first (Christison et al. 1991; Meltzer 1992; Wolkowitz 1993). The use of clozapine in this context is reviewed in Chapter 1 in this volume and by Meltzer (1992). Numerous adjunctive treatments have been investigated in the treatment of schizophrenia, including lithium, carbamazepine, reserpine, benzodiazepines, electroconvulsive therapy, and antidepressants.

In this chapter, I focus on benzodiazepine treatment in patients with schizophrenia; the use of other adjunctive treatments is reviewed elsewhere (Christison et al. 1991; Donaldson et al. 1983; Wolkowitz 1993). As noted in these reviews, no adjunctive treatment benefits all patients; indeed, only a minority respond to any one. A promising area of research is the delineation of biologically distinct subgroups of patients with schizophrenia who may respond preferentially to different classes of adjunctive agents (Wolkowitz et al. 1990).

Rationales for Benzodiazepine Treatment

Response to Stress

Considerable evidence suggests that stressful life events provoke psychotic exacerbations in patients with schizophrenia (Breier et al. 1991b; Norman and Malla 1993a, 1993b; Steinhauser et al. 1991) and that patients with schizophrenia are particularly vulnerable to the effects of stress (Breier et al. 1993; Steinhauser et al. 1991). Clinical observations indicate that patients with schizophrenia respond strongly to changes in level of psychosocial stress (Liddle et al. 1989; Norman and Malla 1993b; Weinberger 1987), and an important objective in the long-term management of patients with schizophrenia is the reduction of environmental stress. According to stress-vulnerability hypotheses, any mechanism that enhances tolerance to stress should reduce the likelihood of expressed symptoms (Steinhauser et al. 1991). Benzodiazepines are clearly effective anxiolytics and may, therefore, secondarily decrease psychotic reactions. Kirkpatrick et al. (1989) and Sovner and Parnell-Sovner (1989) reported that openly administered diazepam and buspirone (a nonbenzodiazepine anxiolytic) attenuated early signs of relapse or minimized stress-induced psychotic exacerbations in some patients with schizophrenia.

Effects on Dopamine Neurotransmission

In addition to having anxiolytic effects, benzodiazepines may have more specific antipsychotic effects via two additional mechanisms. Animal studies have demonstrated that benzodiazepines decrease nigrostriatal dopamine release and turnover (Rastogi et al. 1980; Wood et al. 1982), block stress-induced activations in prefrontal cortical dopamine turnover (Kaneyuki et al. 1991; Lavielle et al. 1978), attenuate acute neuroleptic-induced increases and augment chronic neuroleptic-induced decreases in dopamine turnover (Keller et al. 1976; Singhal et al. 1983), and potentiate the cataleptic effects of neuroleptics (Keller et al. 1976). Thus, benzodiazepine-induced decreases in dopamine release may augment neuroleptic-induced postsynaptic dopamine-receptor blockade, leading to a greater net decrease in dopamine neurotransmission. In a small-scale study of alprazolam augmentation of neuroleptics in patients with treatment-resistant schizophrenia, Wolkowitz et al. (1988) noted that antipsychotic responses were significantly correlated with alprazolam-associated decreases in plasma levels of homovanillic acid, the major dopamine metabolite in humans.

Benzodiazepines exert their principal actions in brain by facilitating γ-aminobutyric acid (GABA) neurotransmission at the benzodiazepine-GABA receptor complex. E. Roberts (1972) and van Kammen (1977) proposed a GABA hypothesis of schizophrenia that postulates inadequate GABA inhibition of dopamine neurotransmission in this illness. Although cerebrospinal fluid and plasma GABA levels have provided inconsistent evidence to support this hypothesis (see Wolkowitz and Pickar 1991), Reynolds et al. (1990) reported a low density of GABA uptake sites in hippocampus samples from autopsied brains of patients with schizophrenia. This deficit was correlated in the left hemisphere with higher than normal dopamine concentrations in the amygdala. Other investigators have observed similar abnormalities in GABA uptake sites (Simpson et al. 1989), GABA receptor binding (Benes et al. 1992), and free GABA levels in brain tissue in patients with schizophrenia (Kutay et al. 1989). It is thus possible that functional impairments in GABA-dopamine interactions during stress are involved in schizophrenic exacerbations; this might explain the efficacy of benzodiazepines in certain patients (Breier et al. 1991b).

The Prefrontal Cortical Dopamine System

Several important dopamine tracts have been identified in the brain, including the nigrostriatal, mesolimbic, and mesoprefrontocortical. Several characteristics differentiate the mesoprefrontocortical tract from the others. In rats, it shows diminished acute and chronic biochemical and electrophysiological response to neuroleptics (Bannon and Roth 1983) and increased sensitivity to stress activation, β-carbolines (benzodiazepine receptor inverse agonists), and benzodiazepines (Deutch et al. 1985; Kaneyuki et al. 1991; Lavielle et al. 1978; Tam and Roth 1985). Alterations in the integrity or function of the stress- and benzodiazepine-sensitive prefrontal cortex may relate to the variability in clinical response to benzodiazepines (Wolkowitz and Pickar 1991; Wolkowitz et al. 1988).

Prefrontal cortical efferents appear to modulate subcortical dopamine responses, particularly during periods of stress. Deutch et al. (1990), for example, found that lesioning the prefrontal cortex rendered dopamine activity in the nucleus accumbens hyperresponsive to stress. Similarly, Scatton et al. (1982) found that frontal cortical ablation in rats resulted in lowered levels of nigral glutamic acid decarboxylase (the enzyme responsible for converting glutamic acid to GABA) and in behaviors consistent with increased striatal dopamine release. These behaviors were reversed by administration of GABAmimetic agents. More recently, Breier et al. (1993) demonstrated that schizophrenic patients with greater prefrontal cortical atrophy (assessed on magnetic resonance image scan) showed enhanced plasma homovanillic acid responses to a metabolic stress challenge. These results are consistent with the possibility that patients with decreased prefrontal cortical volume are particularly sensitive to the dopamine release-stimulating effects of stress and that such patients may also be particularly responsive to benzodiazepine treatment (Wolkowitz and Pickar 1991). Indeed, in a small-scale, preliminary study, Wolkowitz et al. (1988) noted that clinical responders to alprazolam augmentation of neuroleptics showed significantly greater radiographic evidence of prefrontal cortical atrophy than did the clinical nonresponders. Such findings, which could have important implications for the delineation of biologically distinct subgroups of patients with schizophrenia, are undergoing larger-scale replication.

Review of the Literature

Despite these intriguing rationales for benzodiazepine treatment and despite the current widespread use of benzodiazepines in the treatment of schizophrenia (Greenstein et al. 1986; Johnson 1985; Pecknold 1993), the evidence is mixed for the overall efficacy of benzodiazepines in groups of patients with schizophrenia (Wolkowitz et al. 1992). This is likely attributable to the heterogeneous response of patients to these agents. An estimated 30%–50% of patients with schizophrenia respond favorably to benzodiazepine augmentation (Arana et al. 1986; Wolkowitz and Pickar 1991). The average results of any given study, therefore, depend on the proportion of responders versus nonresponders included in the sample (Christison et al. 1991; Wolkowitz et al. 1990). In the following sections, we review the data from double-blind trials of benzodiazepines (used alone or adjunctively) in schizophrenia and consider sources of individual variability in response. Greater detail about the individual studies is provided in a prior review (Wolkowitz and Pickar 1991). We conclude with practical guidelines for clinical management and present several case examples.

Benzodiazepines as Sole Agents

Fourteen double-blind studies examined the efficacy of benzodiazepines, used alone, in the treatment of schizophrenia. Of these, 9 demonstrated some degree of efficacy (*positive* studies: Hankoff et al. 1962; Hekimian and Friedhoff 1967; Jimerson et al. 1982; Lerner et al. 1979; Maculans 1964; Nestoros et al. 1982; Nishikawa et al. 1982; Rao 1964; Smith 1961; *negative* studies: Azima et al. 1962; Gundlach et al. 1966; Holden et al. 1968; Merlis et al. 1962; Stonehill et al. 1966). The more recent studies (post-1975) that employed more rigorous methodologies, diagnostic criteria, and statistical analyses all showed some (generally mild) evidence of positive effects, although 1 examined only the acute (1–24 hours) effects of benzodiazepines (Lerner et al. 1979), and 1 examined only the prolongation of remission (Nishikawa et al. 1982). Among these studies, behavioral improvement was assessed based on a variety of clinical responses. Of the 10 studies that specifically examined improvement in psychosis, 6 demonstrated favorable effects (Jimerson et al. 1982; Lerner et al. 1979; Maculans 1964; Nestoros et al. 1982; Nishikawa et al. 1982; Rao 1964), and 1 of the remaining 4 showed benzodiazepines to be superior to placebo but inferior to neuroleptics (Hekimian and Friedhoff 1967). Therefore, benzodiazepines, even when used alone, may have mild antipsychotic efficacy in some patients.

Benzodiazepines as Adjunctive Agents

Eighteen double-blind studies have examined the efficacy of benzodiazepines used as adjuncts to neuroleptic treatment (Altamura et al. 1987; Barbee et al. 1992; Csernansky et al. 1988; Guz et al. 1972; Hanlon et al. 1969, 1970; Holden et al. 1968; Karson et al. 1982; Kellner et al. 1975; Lingjaerde 1982; Lingjaerde et al. 1979; Marneros 1979; Michaux et al. 1966; Nestoros et al. 1983; Pato et al. 1989; Ruskin et al. 1979; Wolkowitz et al. 1988, 1993). Nine of these studies showed positive effects (Barbee et al. 1992; Guz et al. 1972; Kellner et al. 1975; Lingjaerde 1982; Lingjaerde et al. 1979; Marneros 1979; Nestoros et al. 1983; Wolkowitz et al. 1988, 1993), and 4 indicated mixed or only transiently positive effects (Altamura et al. 1987; Csernansky et al. 1988; Holden et al. 1968; Pato et al. 1989). More than two-thirds of the studies reported after 1975 demonstrated positive results, and 6 of 15 studies that specifically examined antipsychotic effects also demonstrated positive results (Guz et al. 1972; Kellner et al. 1975; Lingjaerde 1982; Lingjaerde et al. 1979; Wolkowitz et al. 1988, 1993).

Two double-blind studies of benzodiazepine augmentation of neuroleptics have been reported since our prior review of this topic (Wolkowitz and Pickar 1991). In the first study, 28 acutely psychotic patients with schizophrenia who were admitted to an emergency psychiatric service were treated with either haloperidol plus placebo or haloperidol plus alprazolam under double-blind conditions for 72 hours (Barbee et al. 1992). Both groups improved significantly; however, the combination-treated group required significantly less neuroleptic and had 56% fewer dystonic reactions. Adjunctive alprazolam was most effective in treating excitement and uncooperativeness.

In the second double-blind study, 42 treatment-resistant patients with schizophrenia or schizoaffective illness ("primarily schizophrenic" subtype, by Research Diagnostic Criteria [Spitzer et al. 1978]) were treated for 4 weeks with either neuroleptics plus placebo or neuroleptics plus alprazolam (mean daily dose, 3.7 mg) (Wolkowitz et al. 1993). Twenty-four of these patients were moderately ill and were largely recruited from outpatient settings; for study purposes, they were hospitalized at an acute inpatient service. The remaining 18 patients were chronically ill, severely treatment-resistant patients who were institutionalized in a state hospital setting. In the moderately ill group, alprazolam augmentation was associated with significant amelioration of positive and negative symptoms of schizophrenia. Decreases in ratings of positive symptoms averaged 22% (versus 6% for placebo), and decreases in ratings of negative symptoms averaged 32% (versus an 8% increase for placebo). The severely ill, treatment-refractory state hospital cohort, however, showed no benefit from alprazolam augmentation.

Factors in Clinical Response

Solitary Versus Adjunctive Treatment

Although benzodiazepines alone may have antipsychotic or tranquilizing efficacy for some patients with schizophrenia, these drugs are clearly less useful than neuroleptics. Therefore, benzodiazepines, when effective, are best used as adjunctive treatments in treatment-resistant patients or used alone in patients who cannot tolerate neuroleptics.

Comparisons of Specific Drugs

The benzodiazepines, and their relative potencies, that have been studied in the treatment of schizophrenia are presented in Table 8–2. There is no clear evidence that specific benzodiazepines differ in their efficacy in schizophrenia (Wolkowitz and Pickar 1991), although Bodkin (1990) suggested that various benzodiazepines (used adjunctively) have different effects on coexisting mood disturbances. High- or intermediate-potency benzodiazepines generally have been associated with more favorable results, but this

Table 8–2. Relative potencies of benzodiazepines studied in the treatment of schizophrenia

Benzodiazepine	Mean dose (mg/day)[a]
Diazepam	22
Chlordiazepoxide	58
Alprazolam	2
Lorazepam	5
Clonazepam	1–5
Estazolam	1.5
Camazepam[b]	40

Note. Only the benzodiazepines studied in the double-blind trials reviewed in this chapter are included in this table. Inclusion here does not imply effectiveness or superiority in the treatment of schizophrenia.
[a]For all drugs except clonazepam, the number shown is the mean of the recommended dose range for the treatment of anxiety (in nonschizophrenic populations); doses for treating schizophrenia may vary. Clonazepam is not listed for this indication, and the numbers shown are the range of doses used in the studies (Altamura et al. 1987; Karson et al. 1982).
[b]Not currently available in the United States.

finding is confounded by the higher doses (corrected for potency) used in those studies. Triazolobenzodiazepines may be mildly superior to other benzodiazepines, at least in the short-term treatment of negative symptoms (Csernansky et al. 1988; Lingjaerde 1985). Further clinical trials to compare triazolobenzodiazepines directly with other high-potency benzodiazepines are required to address this issue.

Onset and Duration of Response

Benzodiazepines may have a rapid onset of therapeutic action. Several investigators have noted beneficial effects of benzodiazepines within the first several hours, days, or weeks of treatment, which is a more rapid time frame than other neuroleptics typically require to reach maximum efficacy (Altamura et al. 1987; Arana et al. 1986; Barbee et al. 1992; Csernansky et al. 1988; Douyon et al. 1989; Guz et al. 1972; Hanlon et al. 1969; Hekimian and Friedhoff 1967; Holden et al. 1968; Kirkpatrick et al. 1989; Lerner et al. 1979; Nestoros et al. 1982; Wolkowitz et al. 1986b, 1988; Yassa et al. 1989). Despite this rapid response, several studies have suggested an early termination of therapeutic effect, often at the fourth week of treatment (Altamura et al. 1987; Arana et al. 1986; Csernansky et al. 1988; Hanlon et al. 1969, 1970; Hekimian and Friedhoff 1967; Holden et al. 1968). Although these studies suggested that patients may become tolerant to the therapeutic effects of benzodiazepines, other studies and case reports noted more long-lasting benefits (Csernansky et al. 1988; Guz et al. 1972; Konafsky and Lindenmayer 1993; Kulik and Wilbur 1986; Nishikawa et al. 1982; Rao 1964; Smith 1961; Wolkowitz et al. 1988, 1989; Yassa et al. 1989). Because this issue is unresolved, several authors have recommended against maintenance benzodiazepine treatment in patients with schizophrenia (Chouinard 1988; Salzman 1988). However, in the first study to address directly the maintenance of response to benzodiazepines, seven patients who had responded favorably to a 4-week trial of alprazolam augmentation of neuroleptics in a double-blind study continued taking neuroleptics plus alprazolam in an open-label, outpatient follow-up study for up to 37 months (mean = 14.3 ± 12.2 months SD) (Turetsky et al. 1993). These patients were compared with another group of six outpatients receiving neuroleptics alone. The patients who received neuroleptics plus alprazolam generally maintained the initial therapeutic effects of alprazolam augmentation through the follow-up period and did not require increasing doses of alprazolam. One patient showed partial behavioral tolerance, and one had alprazolam discontinued because of interdose anxiety symptoms. In several of the patients maintained on adjunctive alprazolam, doses of the concomitant neuroleptics during the follow-up period were decreased. None of the patients maintained on neuroleptics alone showed incremental improvement during the follow-up period, and none sustained decreases in neuroleptic doses. These data indicate the need for a larger-scale, blinded study of the possible role of benzodiazepine maintenance in selected patients. The potential risks of long-term benzodiazepine treatment are discussed later in this chapter, in "Clinical Guidelines and Considerations."

Dose, Plasma Level, and Pharmacokinetic Interactions

The authors of several review articles have noted that higher doses of benzodiazepines appear to be associated with superior responses (Lingjaerde 1985; Nestoros 1980; van Kammen 1977; Wolkowitz and Pickar 1991). Studies reported better responses with higher doses of benzodiazepines, either used alone or as adjunctive treatment, than with lower doses (Table 8–3). Although these data suggest a dose-response relationship, they are not conclusive because few studies have internally assessed dose-response relationships. One open-label study, however, did note greater improvement with lorazepam doses of 2 mg/day or greater compared with lower doses (Cohen and Khan 1987).

Table 8–3. Benzodiazepines: dose response

	Benzodiazepines alone	Adjunctive benzodiazepines
Positive studies	$124^* \pm 103$	$54^* \pm 35$
Negative studies	33 ± 6	22 ± 21

*$P < .05$, compared with negative studies. Doses are in diazepam equivalents (mg/day).

Whereas some studies have found a significant association between plasma benzodiazepine levels and clinical response (Altamura et al. 1987; Csernansky et al. 1988), others have not (Wolkowitz et al. 1988). One study found that serum haloperidol levels were increased in patients receiving a combination of haloperidol and alprazolam compared with patients receiving haloperidol alone, even though the former group received lower doses of haloperidol thus raising the possibility of a pharmacokinetic interaction (Barbee et al. 1992). Other studies, however, found that pharmacokinetic interactions between benzodiazepines and neuroleptics were either clinically insignificant (Douyon et al. 1989) or absent (Wolkowitz et al. 1988).

Response Specificity

Different scenarios for benzodiazepine use in schizophrenia have been investigated (Table 8–4). Studies have suggested a role for adjunctive benzodiazepines in the acute management of psychotic agitation or disruptive behavior. In these situations, benzodiazepines may lead to more rapid tranquilization and may allow the use of lower doses of neuroleptics (Arana et al. 1986; Barbee et al. 1992; Garza-Treviño et al. 1989; Salzman 1988; Salzman et al. 1986), which minimizes neuroleptic side effects (Barbee et al. 1992).

In addition, several studies indicate that benzodiazepines may ameliorate anxiety, hostility, irritability, and even depressive symptoms in patients with schizophrenia (Altamura et al. 1987;

Table 8–4. Scenarios for adjunctive benzodiazepine use in schizophrenia

Rapid control of acute psychotic agitation
Amelioration of anxiety, hostility, irritability, insomnia, and depression in some patients
Amelioration of positive and negative psychotic symptoms in some patients
Acute amelioration of motor disturbances (e.g., catatonia)
Reduction of neuroleptic side effects (e.g., akathisia, tremor, extrapyramidal symptoms)
Possible role in the prophylaxis of stress-induced psychotic exacerbations

Guz et al. 1972; Holden et al. 1968; Jimerson et al. 1982; Kellner et al. 1975; Maculans 1964; Marneros 1979; Nestoros et al. 1982; Pato et al. 1989; Rao 1964). Several studies have also suggested that benzodiazepines may reduce core psychotic symptoms, such as hallucinations, delusions, and thought disorder, in some patients (Guz et al. 1972; Jimerson et al. 1982; Kellner et al. 1975; Lerner et al. 1979; Lingjaerde 1982; Lingjaerde et al. 1979; Nestoros et al. 1982; Pato et al. 1989; Rao 1964; Wolkowitz et al. 1988, 1993). However, in other studies, benzodiazepines had detrimental effects or attenuated the therapeutic effects of neuroleptics in some patients (Arana et al. 1986; Bacher et al. 1986; Dixon et al. 1989; Hanlon et al. 1969, 1970; Jimerson et al. 1982; Lingjaerde 1982; Michaux et al. 1966; Pato et al. 1989). Pato et al. (1989) suggested that the response of psychotic symptoms to benzodiazepines is associated with the response of other symptoms such as anxiety and depression; this suggests a broad distinction between benzodiazepine responders and nonresponders.

Several studies have also suggested that benzodiazepines ameliorate negative symptoms, such as lack of spontaneity, emotional withdrawal, blunted affect, and negativism, in some patients (Csernansky et al. 1988; Holden et al. 1968; Jimerson et al. 1982; Maculans 1964; Nestoros et al. 1982; Wolkowitz et al. 1986b, 1988, 1993). Patients may demonstrate rapid and occasionally striking improvements in social relatedness, spontaneity, and interest in family and social life. Corbett et al. (1993) recently developed an animal model of negative symptoms such as social withdrawal. In the social interaction test in rats, the atypical antipsychotics clozapine and risperidone as well as the benzodiazepine diazepam resulted in significantly increased social interactions. Typical neuroleptic drugs such as haloperidol and chlorpromazine, however, decreased social behaviors during this test.

Finally, benzodiazepines may reduce motor disturbances (e.g., motor unrest, catatonia, akathisia, and other extrapyramidal symptoms) (Altamura et al. 1987; Donlon 1973; Gagrat et al. 1978; Guz et al. 1972; Holden et al. 1968; Lipinski and Cohen 1986; Marneros 1979; Menza and Harris 1989; Michaux et al. 1966; Ruskin et al. 1979). This reduction in motor effects may secondarily reduce psychotic-like symptoms (Lipinski and Cohen 1986; Wolkowitz et al. 1986a).

Variability and Predictors of Response

It is estimated that 30%–50% of patients with schizophrenia respond well to benzodiazepine treatment (Arana et al. 1986; Wolkowitz and Pickar 1991), but no reliable predictors indicate which patients will respond. However, certain studies suggest that patients with more prominent initial psychotic and/or anxiety or panic symptoms or with more severe motor tension, agitation, or retardation respond more favorably to benzodiazepines (Kahn et al. 1988; Kellner et al. 1975; Michaux et al. 1966; Ruskin et al. 1979; Wolkowitz et al. 1988). Chronically ill, severely treatment-refractory patients may show little response (Wolkowitz et al. 1993); conversely, relatively asymptomatic neuroleptic-responsive outpatients or outpatients with postpsychotic depression may respond more poorly to benzodiazepine augmentation or may have difficulty tolerating the sedating side effects (Adan and Siris 1989; Dixon et al. 1989). Adan and Siris (1989) also suggested that inpatients, who have a more stimulating environment, more staff attention, and closer monitoring of dose and side effects, may respond favorably to benzodiazepine augmentation. Biological predictors of treatment responsivity are currently being investigated (Wolkowitz et al. 1988, 1992, 1993).

Clinical Guidelines and Considerations

As with any treatment, the benefits of benzodiazepine treatment must be weighed against the risks. Possible side effects include sedation, ataxia, cognitive impairment, behavioral disinhibition or maniclike behaviors, and even psychotic exacerbation (Arana et al. 1986; Bacher et al. 1986; Dixon et al. 1989; Dorevitch 1991; Hanlon et al. 1969, 1970; Jimerson et al. 1982; Karson et al. 1982; Michaux et al. 1966; Pato et al. 1989; Wolkowitz et al. 1988). In our experience with alprazolam augmentation, approximately 10% of inpatients treated in a research setting developed behavioral disinhibition, which responded to dosage lowering. In the review by Arana et al. (1986), the incidence of arousal and excitation was 34%. The incidence also may be high in outpatients (Dixon et al. 1989; Pato et al. 1989). Therefore, close clinical monitoring of patients is important, especially in outpatient settings (Adan and Siris 1989; Dixon et al. 1989; Pato et al. 1989).

Patients may experience a transient rebound worsening in anxiety, psychotic symptoms, and insomnia following benzodiazepine withdrawal (Jimerson et al. 1982; Karson et al. 1982; K. Roberts and Vass 1986; Wolkowitz et al. 1988). Therefore, benzodiazepines should be tapered gradually, especially following prolonged treatment or treatment with high-potency benzodiazepines with short half-lives. Patients who are likely to be poorly compliant with medication regimens are usually poor candidates for benzodiazepine treatment other than very short-term benzodiazepines.

Furthermore, benzodiazepines may lead to physiological dependence or abuse (Marks 1978; Schmidt et al. 1989; Woods et al. 1988). The risk of abuse in therapeutic settings is considered small, although the risk is higher in patients with histories of drug abuse (Marks 1978; Romach et al. 1991; Schmidt et al. 1989; Woods et al. 1988). Siris (1990) suggested that benzodiazepines may be particularly useful for patients with schizophrenia who abuse substances in an attempt to "self-medicate" anxiety, panic, or negative symptoms. However, in patients who abuse substances, a benzodiazepine trial should not be undertaken trivially and should not be continued unless there is clear therapeutic gain. Most of the studies of benzodiazepine treatment assessed therapeutic effects for less than 8 weeks; data on more prolonged treatment are sparse (Chouinard 1988; Salzman 1988; Turetsky et al. 1993).

Conclusion

The following conclusions are supported by the literature but must remain tentative until more definitive studies are completed:

1. Benzodiazepine response varies considerably among patients; approximately 30%–50% of patients show beneficial effects. Predictors of response are unknown, but patients with acute psychotic symptoms and agitation, anxiety, or panic or patients with motoric disturbances may be most likely to respond. Relatively nonpsychotic outpatients and chronically ill extremely treatment-resistant inpatients may respond more poorly.

2. Benzodiazepines are more effective when used adjunctively but may be mildly effective when used alone in certain patients.
3. The magnitude of therapeutic response to benzodiazepines, when seen, is often modest but may be striking in individual patients.
4. Higher doses of benzodiazepines may be associated with better responses, although therapeutic effects may be seen in the range of commonly prescribed, subsedating doses.
5. Therapeutic effects of benzodiazepines, when seen, may develop rapidly, often within hours, days, or 1–2 weeks. It is reasonable, therefore, to discontinue benzodiazepine treatment after 2 weeks if no response has been seen. This approach minimizes the possibility of deleterious side effects or abuse. Some responsive patients exhibit apparent behavioral tolerance to the therapeutic effects after several weeks, although other patients show longer-lasting responses.
6. Different clinical scenarios exist for the use of benzodiazepines in schizophrenia. Sedation, tranquilization, and reductions in agitation may be the most prominent effects; therefore, benzodiazepines (used adjunctively with neuroleptics) are often useful for the acute management of psychotic agitation or disruptive behavior. In some patients, positive and negative psychotic symptoms are significantly reduced, and certain motor disturbances are diminished. Benzodiazepines may minimize stress-induced exacerbations of psychosis during maintenance treatment in selected patients, but this possibility requires double-blind validation.

Table 8–5 details the procedures used in prior research studies at the National Institute of Mental Health (Wolkowitz et al. 1988) and at the University of California at San Francisco (Wolkowitz et al. 1993) as an example of guidelines for the use of benzodiazepines in schizophrenia. Specific guidelines must obviously be tailored to the specific patient and clinical setting.

Clinical Vignettes

As mentioned earlier in this chapter, clinical response to benzodiazepines is remarkably varied, and improvements, when seen,

Table 8–5. Example of clinical management guidelines for use of benzodiazepines in schizophrenia

1. Start at 0.5 mg qhs (alprazolam or equivalent); increase or decrease dose as tolerated by ≤ 0.5 mg/day (qid dosing for short half-life drugs such as alprazolam) to maximum dose of 5 mg/day. Titrate to subsedating dose.
2. Monitor closely; decrease dose if side effects or disinhibition occurs.
3. Discontinue if no improvement in 2 weeks. Watch for development of tolerance during treatment.
4. Withdraw drug gradually. Observe for rebound symptoms.
5. For outpatients: start low, go slow, perform frequent clinical evaluations.

Note. Guidelines based on National Institute of Mental Health and University of California at San Francisco research protocols.

are often modest. The following two examples of especially good responses portray the type of outcome that is possible.

Case 1

A 30-year-old man with a diagnosis of chronic paranoid schizophrenia had a 6-year history of persistent auditory and visual hallucinations, paranoia, and delusions of thought broadcasting and thought withdrawal. Previous trials of perphenazine, loxapine, and fluphenazine had been only partially successful. Before alprazolam augmentation, he displayed stable and active psychotic symptoms, negativism, and thoughts of self-harm. Alprazolam was added, in a double-blind manner, to his consistent regimen of fluphenazine (30 mg/day), in increasing doses up to 3.5 mg/day. After 1–2 weeks (alprazolam dose 1.5–3.0 mg/day), the patient reported less intrusive hallucinations, and the nurses noted that his functioning was at its best since he was hospitalized. Because the patient became sedated as the dose was increased to 3.5 mg/day, the dose was lowered to 2.0 mg/day. The patient's parents reported a "warmth" in the patient that they had not seen before.

As the dose was further lowered to 1.0 mg/day, his psychotic symptoms returned, and he expressed discouragement and renewed thoughts of self-harm. After alprazolam was discontinued, his symptoms intensified to above prealprazolam levels for 2–3 weeks, after which he returned to his baseline level of severity.

Case 1 demonstrates several points discussed in this chapter. After alprazolam augmentation, this patient showed a clinically significant and fairly rapid reduction in both positive and negative psychotic symptoms and in depression. Relatively higher doses were associated with better response, but the highest dose (3.5 mg/day) was associated with excessive sedation. It was possible to adjust the dose to a subsedating level while maintaining therapeutic benefit. After alprazolam withdrawal, a transient exacerbation of symptoms was observed.

Case 2

A 34-year-old man with a diagnosis of chronic paranoid schizophrenia had been stabilized on a regimen of fluphenazine decanoate, 2 cc im every week but still had persistent paranoid delusions, depression, and suicidality. Adjunctive alprazolam was titrated to a dose of 1.5–1.75 mg/day, in a double-blind manner, at which point the patient reported less paranoia but excessive sedation. He also reported that his suicidal thoughts had disappeared, but he experienced lability of mood, with giggling alternating with sadness. The nursing staff noted that he was more irritable and was having trouble with concentration and memory. After the alprazolam dose was decreased to 1.25 mg/day, he was less sedated and irritable and had no more trouble with memory. He apologized for his earlier paranoia and irritability and said that he now felt less anxious than before he began taking the study drug and, therefore, less paranoid. He reported: "My paranoia is slowed down; I can let go of it and forget about it in a minute or two." After the double-blind trial was completed, the patient was followed on an open-label, outpatient basis with alprazolam doses of 1.0 mg/day (added to his stable fluphenazine regimen). At 8- and 22-month follow-up, the patient maintained the improvements seen initially with double-blind treatment, and the dose of alprazolam remained constant throughout the follow-up period. The patient said: "It keeps me calmer and on track. I have much less temper and don't want to get sore at people. I was more uptight and paranoid before Xanax; it helps me open up a little more with other people."

Case 2 also demonstrates several points discussed in this chapter. As in Case 1, this patient experienced sedation and other side effects, such as memory impairment and mild behavioral disinhibition, on higher doses of alprazolam. However, as in Case 1, slight reductions in dose achieved a therapeutic effect without undue side effects. This patient clearly experienced a stress-reducing effect of the alprazolam and believed this effect was related to his decreased paranoia and his increased social interactiveness. Finally, this patient, who was selected for maintenance treatment based on his favorable initial response to double-blind alprazolam augmentation, continued to show therapeutic effects for at least 22 months, without demonstrating a need for increased doses of alprazolam.

References

Adan F, Siris SG: Trials of adjunctive alprazolam in "negative symptom" patients. Can J Psychiatry 34:326–328, 1989

Altamura AC, Mantero MM, Brunetti M: Clonazepam/haloperidol combination therapy in schizophrenia: a double blind study. Acta Psychiatr Scand 76:702–706, 1987

Arana GW, Ornsteen ML, Kanter F, et al: The use of benzodiazepines for psychotic disorders: a literature review and preliminary clinical findings. Psychopharmacol Bull 22:77–87, 1986

Azima H, Arthurs D, Silver A: The effects of chlordiazepoxide (Librium) in anxiety states. Canadian Psychiatric Association Journal 7:44–50, 1962

Bacher NM, Lewis HA, Field PB: Combined alprazolam and neuroleptic drug in treating schizophrenia. Am J Psychiatry 143:1311–1312, 1986

Bannon MJ, Roth RH: Pharmacology of mesocortical dopamine neurons. Pharmacol Rev 35:53–68, 1983

Barbee JG, Mancuso DM, Freed CR, et al: Alprazolam as a neuroleptic adjunct in the emergency treatment of schizophrenia. Am J Psychiatry 149:506–510, 1992

Benes FM, Vincent SL, Alsterberg G, et al: Increased $GABA_A$ receptor binding in superficial layers of cingulate cortex schizophrenics. J Neurosci 12:924–929, 1992

Bodkin JA: Emerging uses for high-potency benzodiazepines in psychotic disorders. J Clin Psychiatry 51 (suppl 5):41–46, 1990

Breier A, Wolkowitz OM, Doran AR, et al: Neuroleptic responsivity of negative and positive symptoms in schizophrenia. Am J Psychiatry 144:1549–1555, 1987

Breier A, Schreiber JL, Dyer J, et al: National Institute of Mental Health longitudinal study of chronic schizophrenia: prognosis and predictors of outcome. Arch Gen Psychiatry 48:239–246, 1991a

Breier A, Wolkowitz OM, Pickar D: Stress and schizophrenia, in Advances in Neuropsychiatry and Psychopharmacology, Vol 1: Schizophrenia Research. Edited by Tamminga CA, Schulz SC. New York, Raven, 1991b, pp 141–152

Breier A, Davis OR, Buchanan RW, et al: Effects of metabolic perturbation on plasma homovanillic acid in schizophrenia: relationship to prefrontal cortex volume. Arch Gen Psychiatry 50:541–550, 1993

Chouinard G: The use of benzodiazepines in the treatment of manic-depressive illness. Can J Psychiatry 49 (suppl):15–19, 1988

Christison GW, Kirch DG, Wyatt RJ: When symptoms persist: choosing among alternative somatic treatments for schizophrenia. Schizophr Bull 17:217–245, 1991

Cohen S, Khan A: Adjunctive benzodiazepines in acute schizophrenia. Neuropsychobiology 18:9–12, 1987

Corbett R, Hartman H, Kerman LL, et al: Effects of atypical antipsychotic agents on social behavior in rodents. Pharmacol Biochem Behav 45:9–17, 1993

Crow TJ: Positive and negative schizophrenic symptoms and the role of dopamine. Br J Psychiatry 137:383–386, 1980

Csernansky JG, Riney SJ, Lombrozo L, et al: Double-blind comparison of alprazolam, diazepam and placebo for the treatment of negative schizophrenic symptoms. Arch Gen Psychiatry 45:655–659, 1988

Davis JM: Antipsychotic drugs, in Comprehensive Textbook of Psychiatry, Vol 3. Edited by Kaplan HI, Freedman AM, Sadock BJ. Baltimore, MD, Williams & Wilkins, 1980, pp 2257–2289

Deutch AY, Tam SY, Roth RH: Footshock and conditioned stress increase 3,4-dihydroxphenylacetic acid (DOPAC) in the ventral tegmental area but not substantia nigra. Brain Res 333:143–146, 1985

Deutch AY, Clark WA, Roth RH: Prefrontal cortical dopamine depletion enhances the responsiveness of mesolimbic dopamine neurons to stress. Brain Res 521:311–315, 1990

Dixon L, Weiden PJ, Frances AJ, et al: Alprazolam intolerance in stable schizophrenic outpatients. Psychopharmacol Bull 25:213–214, 1989

Donaldson SR, Gelenberg AJ, Baldessarini RJ: The pharmacologic treatment of schizophrenia: a progress report. Schizophr Bull 9:504–527, 1983

Donlon PT: The therapeutic use of diazepam for akathisia. Psychosomatics 14:222–225, 1973

Dorevitch A: Mania associated with clonazepam. Ann Pharmacother 25:938–939, 1991

Douyon R, Angrist B, Peselow E, et al: Neuroleptic augmentation with alprazolam: clinical effects and pharmacokinetic correlates. Am J Psychiatry 146:231–234, 1989

Gagrat D, Hamilton J, Belmaker RH: Intravenous diazepam in the treatment of neuroleptic-induced acute dystonia and akathisia. Am J Psychiatry 135:1232–1233, 1978

Garza-Treviño ES, Hollister LE, Overall JE, et al: Efficacy of combinations of intramuscular antipsychotics and sedative-hypnotics for control of psychotic agitation. Am J Psychiatry 146:1598–1601, 1989

Greenstein RA, Welz WKR, Weisbrot M: Benzodiazepines in schizophrenia (letter). Psychosomatics 27:799, 1986

Gundlach R, Engelhardt DM, Hankoff L, et al: A double-blind outpatient study of diazepam (Valium) and placebo. Psychopharmacologia 9:81–92, 1966

Guz L, Moraea R, Sartoretto JN: The therapeutic effects of lorazepam in psychotic patients treated with haloperidol: a double-blind study. Current Therapeutic Research 14:767–774, 1972

Hankoff LD, Rudorfer L, Paley HM: A reference study of ataraxics: a two-week double blind outpatient evaluation. The Journal of New Drugs 2:173–178, 1962

Hanlon TE, Ota KY, Agallianos DD, et al: Combined drug treatment of newly hospitalized, acutely ill psychiatric patients. Diseases of the Nervous System 30:104–116, 1969

Hanlon TE, Ota KY, Kurland AA: Comparative effects of fluphenazine, fluphenazine-chlordiazepoxide and fluphenazine-imipramine. Diseases of the Nervous System 31:171–177, 1970

Hekimian LJ, Friedhoff AJ: A controlled study of placebo, chlordiazepoxide and chlorpromazine with thirty male schizophrenic patients. Diseases of the Nervous System 28:675–678, 1967

Holden JMC, Itil TM, Keskiner A, et al: Thioridazine and chlordiazepoxide, alone and combined, in the treatment of chronic schizophrenia. Compr Psychiatry 9:633–634, 1968

Jimerson DC, van Kammen DP, Post RM, et al: Diazepam in schizophrenia: a preliminary double-blind trial. Am J Psychiatry 139:489–491, 1982

Johnson DAW: Antipsychotic medication: clinical guidelines for maintenance therapy. J Clin Psychiatry 46:6–15, 1985

Kahn JP, Puertollano MA, Schane MD, et al: Adjunctive alprazolam for schizophrenia with panic anxiety: clinical observation and pathogenic implications. Am J Psychiatry 145:742–744, 1988

Kaneyuki H, Yokoo H, Tsuda A, et al: Psychological stress increases dopamine turnover selectively in mesoprefrontal dopamine neurons of rats: reversal by diazepam. Brain Res 557:154–161, 1991

Karson CN, Weinberger DR, Bigelow L, et al: Clonazepam treatment of chronic schizophrenia: negative results in a double-blind, placebo-controlled trial. Am J Psychiatry 139:1627–1628, 1982

Keller HH, Schaffner R, Haefely W: Interaction of benzodiazepines with neuroleptics at central dopamine neurons. Naunyn Schmiedebergs Arch Pharmacol 294:1–7, 1976

Kellner R, Wilson RM, Muldawer MD, et al: Anxiety in schizophrenia: the response to chlordiazepoxide in an intensive design study. Arch Gen Psychiatry 32:1246–1254, 1975

Kirkpatrick B, Buchanan RW, Waltrip RW, et al: Diazepam treatment of early symptoms of schizophrenic relapse. J Nerv Ment Dis 177:52–53, 1989

Konafsky D, Lindenmayer JP: Relapse following lorazepam withdrawal (letter to the editor). Am J Psychiatry 150:348–349, 1993

Kulik FA, Wilbur R: High dose alprazolam in schizophrenia. J Clin Psychopharmacol 6:191–192, 1986

Kutay FZ, Pögün S, Hariri NI, et al: Free amino acid level determinations in normal and schizophrenic brain. Prog Neuropsychopharmacol Biol Psychiatry 13:119–126, 1989

Lavielle S, Tassin J, Thierry A, et al: Blockade by benzodiazepines of the selective high increase in dopamine turnover induced by stress in mesocortical dopaminergic neurons of the rat. Brain Res 168:585–594, 1978

Lerner Y, Lwow E, Levitin A, et al: Acute high-dose parenteral haloperidol treatment of psychosis. Am J Psychiatry 136:1061–1064, 1979

Liddle PF, Barnes TRE, Morris D, et al: Three syndromes in chronic schizophrenia. Br J Psychiatry 155 (suppl 7):119–122, 1989

Lingjaerde O: Effect of the benzodiazepine derivative estazolam in patients with auditory hallucinations: a multicentre double-blind, crossover study. Acta Psychiatr Scand 65:339–354, 1982

Lingjaerde O: Antipsychotic effect of the benzodiazepines, in Antipsychotics. Edited by Burrows GD, Norman TR, Davies B. Amsterdam, Elsevier, 1985, pp 163–172

Lingjaerde O, Engstrand E, Ellingsen P, et al: Antipsychotic effect of diazepam when given in addition to neuroleptics in chronic psychotic patients: a double-blind clinical trial. Current Therapeutic Research 26:505–514, 1979

Lipinski JF, Cohen BM: Alprazolam-neuroleptic combination in schizophrenia (letter). Am J Psychiatry 143:1501–1502, 1986

Maculans GA: Comparison of diazepam, chlorprothixene and chlorpromazine in chronic schizophrenic patients. Diseases of the Nervous System 25:164–168, 1964

Marks J: The Benzodiazepines: Use, Overuse, Misuse, Abuse. Baltimore, MD, University Park Press, 1978

Marneros A: Anxiolytische zusatzbehandlung bei den affektbetonten schizophrenien. Therapiewoche 29:7533–7538, 1979

McDermott, Sautter FJ, Garver DL: Heterogeneity of schizophrenia: relationship to latency of neuroleptic response. Psychiatry Res 37:97–103, 1991

Meltzer HY: Treatment of the neuroleptic-nonresponsive schizophrenic patient. Schizophr Bull 18:515–542, 1992

Menza MA, Harris D: Benzodiazepines and catatonia: an overview. Biol Psychiatry 26:842–846, 1989

Merlis S, Turner WJ, Krumholz W: A double-blind comparison of diazepam, chlordiazepoxide and chlorpromazine in psychotic patients. Journal of Neuropsychiatry 3 (suppl 1):S133–S138, 1962

Michaux MH, Kurland AA, Afallianos DD: Chlorpromazine-chlordiazepoxide and chlorpromazine-imipramine treatment of newly hospitalized, acutely ill psychiatry patients. Current Therapeutic Research 8:117–152, 1966

Nestoros JN: Benzodiazepines in schizophrenia: a need for reassessment. International Pharmacopsychiatry 15:171–179, 1980

Nestoros JN, Suranyi-Cadotte BE, Spees RC, et al: Diazepam in high doses is effective in schizophrenia. Prog Neuropsychopharmacol Biol Psychiatry 6:513–516, 1982

Nestoros JN, Nair NPV, Pulman JR, et al: High doses of diazepam improve neuroleptic-resistant chronic schizophrenic patients. Psychopharmacology (Berl) 81:42–47, 1983

Nishikawa T, Tsuda A, Tanaka M, et al: Prophylactic effect of neuroleptics in symptom-free schizophrenics. Psychopharmacology (Berl) 77:301–304, 1982

Norman RMG, Malla AK: Stressful life events and schizophrenia, I: a review of the research. Br J Psychiatry 162:161–166, 1993a

Norman RMG, Malla AK: Stressful life events and schizophrenia, II: conceptual and methodological issues. Br J Psychiatry 162:166–174, 1993b

Pato CN, Wolkowitz OM, Rapaport M, et al: Benzodiazepine augmentation of neuroleptic treatment in patients with schizophrenia. Psychopharmacol Bull 25:263–266, 1989

Pecknold JC: Survey of the adjuvant use of benzodiazepines for treating outpatients with schizophrenia. J Psychiatry Neurosci 18:82–84, 1993

Pickar D: Pharmacotherapeutic approaches to schizophrenia, in Psychopharmacology Consultation. Edited by Jimerson DC, Docherty JP. Washington, DC, American Psychiatric Press, 1986, pp 71–103

Pickar D: Perspectives on a time-dependent model of neuroleptic action. Schizophr Bull 14:255–268, 1988

Rao AV: A controlled trial with "Valium" in some psychiatric disorders. Indian Journal of Psychiatry 4:188–192, 1964

Rastogi RB, Lapierre YD, Singhal RL, et al: Evidence for involvement of dopamine in the action of diazepam: potentiation of haloperidol and chlorpromazine action in the brain. Adv Biochem Psychopharmacol 24:283–289, 1980

Reynolds GP, Czudek C, Andrews HB: Deficit and hemispheric asymmetry of GABA uptake sites in the hippocampus in schizophrenia. Biol Psychiatry 27:1038–1044, 1990

Roberts E: An hypothesis suggesting that there is a defect in the GABA system in schizophrenia. Neuroscience Research Progress Bulletin 10:468–483, 1972

Roberts K, Vass N: Schneiderian first-rank symptoms caused by benzodiazepine withdrawal. Br J Psychiatry 148:593–594, 1986

Romach MK, Busto UE, Sobell LC, et al: Long-term alprazolam use: abuse, dependence or treatment? Psychopharmacol Bull 27:391–395, 1991

Ruskin P, Averbukh I, Belmaker RH, et al: Benzodiazepines in chronic schizophrenia. Biol Psychiatry 14:557–558, 1979

Salzman C: Use of benzodiazepines to control disruptive behavior in inpatients. J Clin Psychiatry 49:13–15, 1988

Salzman C, Green AI, Rodriguez-Villa F, et al: Benzodiazepines combined with neuroleptics for management of severe disruptive behavior. Psychosomatics 27:17–21, 1986

Scatton B, Worms P, Lloyd KG, et al: Cortical modulation of striatal function. Brain Res 232:331–334, 1982

Schmidt LG, Grohmann R, Muller-Oerlinghausen B, et al: Prevalence of benzodiazepine abuse and dependence in psychiatric inpatients with different nosology. Br J Psychiatry 154:839–843, 1989

Simpson MDC, Slater P, Deakin JFW, et al: Reduced GABA uptake sites in the temporal lobe in schizophrenia. Neurosci Lett 107:211–215, 1989

Singhal RL, Rastogi RB, Laierre YD: Diazepam potentiates the effect of neuroleptics on behavioral activity as well as dopamine and norepinephrine turnover: do benzodiazepines have antipsychotic potency? J Neural Transm Gen Sect 56:127–138, 1983

Siris SG: Pharmacological treatment of substance-abusing schizophrenic patients. Schizophr Bull 16:111–122, 1990

Smith ME: A clinical study of chlorpromazine and chlordiazepoxide. Conn Med 25:153–157, 1961

Sovner R, Parnell-Sovner N: Use of buspirone in the treatment of schizophrenia. J Clin Psychopharmacol 9:61–62, 1989

Spitzer RL, Endicott J, Robins E: Research Diagnostic Criteria: rationale and reliability. Arch Gen Psychiatry 35:773 782, 1978

Steinhauser SR, Zubin J, Condray R, et al: Electrophysiological and behavioral signs of attentional disturbance in schizophrenics and their siblings, in Advances in Neuropsychiatry and Psychopharmacology, Vol I: Schizophrenia Research. Edited by Tamminga CA, Schulz SC. New York, Raven, 1991, pp 169–180

Stonehill E, Lee H, Ban TA: A comparative study with benzodiazepines in chronic psychotic patients. Diseases of the Nervous System 27:411–413, 1966

Tam SY, Roth RH: Selective increase in dopamine metabolism in the prefrontal cortex by the anxiogenic beta-carboline FG-7142. Biochem Pharmacol 34:1595–1598, 1985

Turetsky NG, Wolkowitz OM, Reus VI: Benzodiazepine maintenance in schizophrenia. Paper presented at the annual meeting of the American Psychiatric Association, San Francisco, CA, May 1993

van Kammen DP: gamma-Aminobutyric acid (GABA) and the dopamine hypothesis of schizophrenia. Am J Psychiatry 134:138–143, 463–464, 1977

Weinberger DR: Implications of normal brain development in the pathogenesis of schizophrenia. Arch Gen Psychiatry 44:660–669, 1987

Wolkowitz OM: Rational polypharmacy in schizophrenia. Annals of Clinical Psychiatry 5:79–90, 1993

Wolkowitz OM, Pickar D: Benzodiazepines in the treatment of schizophrenia: a review and reappraisal. Am J Psychiatry 148:714–726, 1991

Wolkowitz OM, Pickar D, Doran AR, et al: Alprazolam-neuroleptic combination in schizophrenia: Dr. Wolkowitz and associates reply. Am J Psychiatry 143:1501–1502, 1986a

Wolkowitz OM, Pickar D, Doran AR, et al: Combination alprazolam-neuroleptic treatment of the positive and negative symptoms of schizophrenia. Am J Psychiatry 143:85–87, 1986b

Wolkowitz OM, Breier A, Doran AR, et al: Alprazolam augmentation of the antipsychotic effects of fluphenazine in schizophrenic patients: preliminary results. Arch Gen Psychiatry 45:664–671, 1988

Wolkowitz OM, Reus VI, Breier A, et al: Alprazolam-neuroleptic treatment in schizophrenia (abstract). Schizophr Res 2:215, 1989

Wolkowitz OM, Bartko JJ, Pickar D: Drug trials and heterogeneity in schizophrenia: the mean is not the end. Biol Psychiatry 28:1021–1025, 1990

Wolkowitz OM, Turetsky N, Reus VI, et al: Benzodiazepine augmentation of neuroleptics in treatment-resistant schizophrenia. Psychopharmacol Bull 28:291–295, 1992

Wolkowitz OM, Harris D, Turetsky NG, et al: Alprazolam-neuroleptic treatment of schizophrenia. Paper presented at the annual meeting of the American Psychiatric Association, San Francisco, CA, May 1993

Wood PL, Etienne P, Samarthji L, et al: GABAergic regulation of nigrostriatal neurons: coupling of benzodiazepine and GABA receptors. Prog Neuropsychopharmacol Biol Psychiatry 6:471–474, 1982

Woods JH, Katz JL, Winger G: Use and abuse of benzodiazepines: issues relevant to prescribing. JAMA 260:3476–3480, 1988

Wyatt RJ: Neuroleptics and the natural course of schizophrenia. Schizophr Bull 17:325–351, 1991

Yassa R, Nastase C, Belzile L: Lorazepam as an adjunct in the treatment of auditory hallucinations in a schizophrenic patient (letter). J Clin Psychopharmacol 9:386, 1989

CHAPTER 9

Treating Negative Symptoms: Pharmacological Strategies

Robert W. Buchanan, M.D.
Martin Brandes, M.D.
Alan Breier, M.D.

The development of effective pharmacological strategies for the treatment of the negative symptoms of schizophrenia is a major challenge facing the field of psychiatry. Two major factors provide the impetus for developing effective treatments. First, negative symptoms tend to show a limited range of response to traditional neuroleptics and persist after the successful treatment of positive psychotic symptoms (Carpenter and Conley 1991). Second, negative symptoms commonly underlie the social and occupational impairments that characterize a significant proportion of patients with chronic schizophrenia. These impairments are often a major factor in preventing patients from leaving the hospital and becoming integrated into the community.

In this chapter, we review the differential diagnosis of negative symptoms (i.e., the differentiation of primary from secondary negative symptoms); the treatment of secondary negative symptoms; and the use of dopamine agonists, noradrenergic and serotonergic agents, anticholinergics, and atypical antipsychotics for the treatment of primary negative symptoms.

Differential Diagnosis and Treatment of Secondary Negative Symptoms

The concept of *negative symptoms* has a long history (Berrios 1985). The term was originally applied in the context of neurological disorders and designated a loss of normal function. The concept of negative symptoms in schizophrenia is derived from Kraepelin's description of personality dissolution in patients with schizophrenia: "the result of this process is emotional dullness, failure of mental activities, loss of mastery over volition, of endeavor, and of ability for independent action" (Kraepelin 1919, p. 74). Over the years, multiple conceptual models have been developed to investigate negative symptoms (Andreasen and Olsen 1982; Carpenter et al. 1988; Crow 1985; Strauss et al. 1974). These models have differed in their emphasis on the role of negative symptoms as a defining feature of schizophrenic subtypes (Andreasen and Olsen 1982; Crow 1985) versus negative symptoms representing symptom complexes with a discrete etiopathophysiology (Carpenter and Buchanan 1989; Carpenter et al. 1988; Strauss et al. 1974). There is now considerable evidence from factor analytic studies that negative symptoms represent an independent cluster of symptoms that can be differentiated from other schizophrenic symptoms (R. W. Buchanan and Carpenter 1994). These studies support the inclusion of affective flattening, alogia, avolition, anhedonia, and asociality as negative symptoms, and it is these symptoms that are emphasized in the evaluation of the effectiveness of pharmacological approaches for treating negative symptoms.

Negative symptoms can either be primary and represent core features of schizophrenia (Carpenter et al. 1988) or secondary to positive psychotic symptoms, side effects of antipsychotic medication, depression or anxiety, or environmental deprivation (Carpenter et al. 1985; Wing and Brown 1970). The differentiation between primary and secondary negative symptoms is of critical importance because treatment approaches vary greatly for the different types of negative symptoms (Carpenter and Conley 1991; Carpenter et al. 1985). Specific pharmacological interventions are available for negative symptoms secondary to psychosis, antipsychotic side effects, and dysphoric affects. These are briefly reviewed in the following sections.

Negative Symptoms Secondary to Psychotic Symptoms

Exacerbations of psychotic symptoms are commonly associated with increases in negative symptoms. The increases in negative symptoms may be related to 1) disorganization of the patient's psychic functions; 2) psychotic preoccupation with idiosyncratic subjective experiences, leading to a reduced ability to interact with the environment; and 3) the use of emotional and social withdrawal as a defensive maneuver to minimize external stimuli and reduce the demand on a patient's disorganized cognitive functions (Carpenter et al. 1985). The paranoid patient's withdrawal from the external environment in response to his or her paranoid delusions is a common example of this latter phenomenon.

Treatment of the underlying psychotic symptoms would be expected to alleviate negative symptoms secondary to psychosis (S. C. Goldberg 1985). It is most critical to ensure that the patient is receiving an adequate trial of neuroleptic drug. If the patient does not respond to adequate neuroleptic treatment, then the use of other typical or atypical antipsychotics is indicated.

Negative Symptoms Secondary to Antipsychotic Medication

Traditional neuroleptic treatment is often associated with the development of side effects that may mimic negative symptoms. Of particular relevance to the treatment of negative symptoms are extrapyramidal side effects (EPS) (e.g., akinesia and masked facies) and sedation. Neuroleptics may also cause dysphoria and, subsequent to the induction of dysphoria, anhedonia.

In addition to EPS and sedation, neuroleptic treatment may produce secondary negative symptoms by decreasing the level of activity of mesocortical dopaminergic neurons projecting to the prefrontal cortex (E. Goldberg 1985). The decreased mesocortical dopaminergic activity would result in symptoms analogous to negative symptoms, including apathy, lack of spontaneity, and impaired affective arousal.

Available pharmacological treatments for negative symptoms secondary to neuroleptic side effects include 1) anticholinergic agents, 2) neuroleptic dosage reduction, 3) use of a different neuroleptic, and 4) neuroleptic discontinuation in the context of a targeted pharmacological approach (Carpenter and Conley 1991). In considering either neuroleptic reduction or discontinuation, the merits of each approach must be balanced against the increased risk of psychotic symptom exacerbation. The decision to use a different neuroleptic usually involves switching a patient from a high-potency agent (e.g., fluphenazine or haloperidol) to a low-potency agent (e.g., thioridazine or chlorpromazine). The high-potency agents tend to be associated with an increased risk for development of EPS, whereas the low-potency agents are more likely to be associated with sedation. Clozapine, an atypical antipsychotic, is an alternative treatment option to traditional neuroleptics for patients who are especially prone to developing EPS, but it is also associated with an increased risk of sedation (Baldessarini and Frankenburg 1991).

Negative Symptoms Secondary to Dysphoric Affect

Symptoms of depression and anxiety occur frequently in patients with schizophrenia. Anhedonia, apathy, loss of interests, and decreased speech and social drive are characteristic of both dysphoric states and negative symptoms. These symptoms may be a direct manifestation of the illness; an indirect manifestation of the illness (e.g., a response to the decreased capacity for coping with stress); a response to having a major illness and associated functional impairments; or, as mentioned previously, a result of neuroleptic treatment (e.g., dysphoria, akathisia). Anxiety and depressive symptoms may be difficult to recognize in patients with schizophrenia because they have a decreased ability to integrate and verbalize their inner experiences and feelings (Carpenter et al. 1985).

Antidepressants, when used as an adjunctive treatment, can be effective in ameliorating depressive symptoms in patients with schizophrenia (A. N. Singh et al. 1978; Siris et al. 1987). Reductions in depressive symptoms may be associated with reductions in negative symptom ratings (Goff et al. 1990; Silver and Nassar 1992). The use of antidepressants in the treatment of negative symptoms is discussed in further detail later in this chapter in the

"Dopamine Agonists," "Noradrenergic Agents," and "Serotonergic Agents" sections.

Similarly, benzodiazepines have been shown to decrease anxiety symptoms and psychotic symptoms in patients with schizophrenia (Csernansky et al. 1984; Douyon et al. 1989; Herrera et al. 1991; Lingjaerde et al. 1979; Nestoros et al. 1982, 1983; Wolkowitz et al. 1986, 1988). In the majority of these studies, benzodiazepines were also observed to have a beneficial effect on negative symptoms (Csernansky et al. 1984; Douyon et al. 1989; Nestoros et al. 1982, 1983; Wolkowitz et al. 1986, 1988). In contrast, four studies failed to document a therapeutic effect of benzodiazepines for negative symptoms (Adan and Siris 1989; Csernansky et al. 1988; Herrera et al. 1991; Lingjaerde et al. 1979). In the double-blind study by Csernansky et al. (1988), benzodiazepines did not reduce positive, affective, or negative symptoms. This study had, by far, the largest sample of any of the studies examining benzodiazepine efficacy. Their results support the interpretation that the beneficial effect of benzodiazepines on negative symptoms is associated with the benzodiazepines' effect on either positive and/or affective symptoms.

Pharmacological Treatment of Negative Symptoms

The negative symptoms that persist after differential diagnosis and treatment most likely represent primary, enduring negative or *deficit* symptoms (Carpenter et al. 1988). The lack of adequate response of primary negative symptoms to traditional neuroleptics has led to the development of alternative pharmacological strategies. However, the ability to evaluate the efficacy of these alternative treatments for primary negative symptoms is limited by several methodological factors. The majority of studies fail to differentiate primary from secondary negative symptoms and/or fail to assess the effect of potential confounding variables (i.e., concurrent changes in level of psychotic, extrapyramidal, or dysphoric symptoms) on observed changes in negative symptoms. Second, the majority of studies have used proxy rather than direct measures of negative symptoms. The failure to attend to these methodological variables limits the ability to evaluate the efficacy of the proposed treatment for primary negative symptoms. Consequently, all studies demonstrating beneficial effects should be considered preliminary until the proposed agent is evaluated in a more methodologically rigorous manner.

We review the following pharmacological approaches: dopamine agonists; noradrenergic and serotonergic agents; anticholinergics; and atypical antipsychotics, including clozapine, risperidone, and remoxipride. We discuss the relative merits and limitations of each approach, with particular emphasis on the methodological issues discussed above.

Dopamine Agonists

The rationale for the use of dopamine agonists for the treatment of negative symptoms is derived from reformulations of the dopamine hypothesis (Davis et al. 1991; Weinberger 1987). These reformulations have posited that schizophrenia is characterized, in part, by decreased mesocortical dopaminergic activity in the prefrontal cortex and that this decreased activity results in the production of negative symptoms. Thus, agents that increase the level of dopamine activity in the prefrontal cortex would be hypothesized to ameliorate negative symptomatology.

L-Dopa is a dopamine precursor that is thought to increase the level of dopaminergic activity by increasing dopamine synthesis. Interest in the use of L-dopa for the treatment of negative symptoms was stimulated by the results of an early study that demonstrated beneficial effects of a single-dose infusion of L-dopa on emotional withdrawal and sense of well-being (Bruno and Bruno 1966). In an open-label trial, Ogura and colleagues (1976) found L-dopa to have mild to moderate effects on both positive and negative symptoms.

Three double-blind studies were conducted to examine the efficacy of L-dopa as an adjunctive treatment to neuroleptics for negative symptoms. Gerlach and Luhdorf (1975) reported that L-dopa/benserazide (a peripheral decarboxylase inhibitor) resulted in significant improvements in the Brief Psychiatric Rating Scale (BPRS; Overall and Gorham 1962) total score and in the BPRS anergia factor, a commonly used proxy for negative symptoms composed of the following items: emotional withdrawal, blunted affect, and psychomotor retardation. Patients also experienced mild improvement in EPS. F. H. Buchanan et al. (1975) found that patients who received L-dopa felt more alive and energetic, but there were no significant rating scale improvements. Finally, Kay and Opler (1985–1986) used a double-blind, placebo-controlled reversal design to assess the effect of L-dopa/carbidopa in a neuroleptic-nonresponsive patient with severe negative symptoms. They found that negative symptoms significantly improved, independent of any change in positive symptoms.

A major concern about the use of L-dopa for the treatment of negative symptoms is that it may exacerbate positive symptoms. Angrist et al. (1973) reported that L-dopa, administered to patients with schizophrenia who were withdrawn from neuroleptic treatment, worsened preexisting psychotic symptoms. However, Alpert et al. (1978), in a double-blind comparison of L-dopa and chlorpromazine, found that L-dopa did not exacerbate psychotic symptoms. In addition, L-dopa has not been shown to cause exacerbations of psychotic symptoms when used as an adjunctive treatment to antipsychotics (F. H. Buchanan et al. 1975; Gerlach and Luhdorf 1975; Kay and Opler 1985–1986).

D-Amphetamine causes dopamine release and blocks dopamine reuptake. The combination of these two properties results in enhanced dopaminergic activity. Three of the four studies that have examined the effect of D-amphetamine on negative symptoms have focused on the acute response of negative symptoms to single D-amphetamine infusions. Angrist et al. (1980) reported that the BPRS anergia factor worsened after D-amphetamine infusion to schizophrenic inpatients, with the change being primarily restricted to worsening of the emotional withdrawal item, which worsened secondarily to increased positive symptoms. In a second study, Angrist et al. (1982) administered D-amphetamine to outpatients with chronic schizophrenia with predominant negative symptoms. They found that D-amphetamine led to a significant improvement in the BPRS anergia factor (minus the emotional withdrawal item). In both studies, the patients had been withdrawn from neuroleptics. van Kammen and Boronow (1988) administered D-amphetamine to patients while on and off pimozide, a selective D_2 antagonist. They found that D-amphetamine significantly decreased BPRS anergia factor scores in drug-free patients with schizophrenia but that this effect was attenuated when the patients were treated with pimozide.

In the only long-term trial of D-amphetamine, Cesarec and Nyman (1985) reported that D-amphetamine given openly, either as an adjunctive treatment or alone, resulted in a mixed pattern of negative symptom responsiveness. Of 17 patients with negative symptoms, 9 patients showed varied degrees of improvement; 3 patients had no change in negative symptoms; and 5 patients worsened, but 4 of the 5 were not receiving concurrent neuroleptics. These latter patients also exhibited worsening of other aspects of their illness.

Mazindol blocks dopamine reuptake at the dopamine transporter site. Seibyl and colleagues (1991, 1992) presented preliminary data that mazindol may decrease negative symptomatology. They found that changes in negative symptoms occurred independently of changes in positive symptoms but that there were concurrent reductions in the level of EPS.

Bromocriptine is an ergot alkaloid with dopamine agonist activity. Two series of case reports provide conflicting data on the efficacy of bromocriptine. King (1978) reported that bromocriptine had no effect on negative symptoms in 2 chronically ill patients withdrawn from neuroleptics. In contrast, Levi-Minzi et al. (1991) found that bromocriptine, when added to neuroleptics, resulted in a marked reduction in negative symptoms in 6 of 20 patients. Bromocriptine's beneficial effect was maintained for up to 9 years. The efficacy of bromocriptine for negative symptoms has also been evaluated in two double-blind studies. Gattaz et al. (1989) examined the effects of low-dose bromocriptine in schizophrenic inpatients and did not find a significant effect for bromocriptine on negative symptoms. In contrast, Wolf et al. (1992) reported that bromocriptine treatment resulted in a significant reduction in the BPRS anergia factor score. However, the reduction in the BPRS anergia factor corresponded to significant reductions in positive symptoms.

Monoamine oxidase is one of the principal enzymes involved in the conversion of dopamine to its metabolites, and its inhibition would be hypothesized to increase dopamine activity. However, monoamine oxidase is also involved in the conversion of norepinephrine to its metabolites. Therefore, if monoamine oxidase inhibitors (MAOIs) are effective for the treatment of negative symptoms, they also may be exerting their therapeutic effect through the noradrenergic system. Two studies have examined the effect of MAOIs on negative symptoms. Tranylcypromine, a nonselective MAOI, was shown to reduce levels of BPRS anergia factor items significantly (Bucci 1987). The reduction in these items corresponded to changes in the BPRS total score and depression item. Perenyi et al. (1992), in an open study, found that L-deprenyl, a selective MAOI-B that may also have direct dopamine agonist activities, reduced negative symptom levels in the absence of changes in positive or depressive symptoms.

Partial dopamine agonists have affinity for both autoreceptors and postsynaptic receptors. Their pharmacological action is dependent on the concentration of the drug at the receptor (at low concentrations they act as agonists, and at high concentrations they act as antagonists), and the relative affinity of the drug for the two types of receptors. Two partial agonists have been examined in open clinical trials: OPC-4392 (Gerbaldo et al. 1988) and terguride (Olbrich and Schanz 1988). In both studies, the partial agonists were found to be effective in reducing levels of negative symptoms. However, Gerbaldo et al. (1988) reported that the reduction in negative symptoms, as measured by the BPRS anergia factor, coincided with reductions in positive symptoms, whereas Olbrich and Schanz (1988, 1991) found terguride to reduce negative symptoms, as assessed by the Scale for the Assessment of Negative Symptoms (SANS; Andreasen 1981), without any change in positive symptoms.

Summary. The results of the dopamine agonist treatment studies argue, at the least, for the continued investigation of these agents for the treatment of negative symptoms. The results provide consistent evidence that a wide range of agents is effective in reducing the level of negative symptoms. However, the majority of studies are characterized by the following methodological limitations: 1) small sample sizes, 2) proxy measures used to assess negative symptoms, and 3) failure to discriminate primary from secondary negative symptoms. In addition, a large number of the reports are either case reports or open trials. Because of these methodological limitations, it cannot be determined whether dopamine agonists are effective treatment for primary negative symptoms or are limited to the alleviation of secondary negative symptoms.

Noradrenergic Agents

Extensive interactions occur between noradrenergic and dopaminergic systems in the prefrontal cortex. Specifically, dopamine afferents have been shown to modulate the sensitivity of cortical postsynaptic β-adrenergic receptors; noradrenergic neurons control, in part, the sensitivity of cortical D_1 receptors; and stimulation of cortical α_1-adrenergic receptors inhibits cortical transmission at D_1 receptors (Tassin 1992). Moreover, norepinephrine levels have been associated with the level of negative symptoms in schizophrenia. In acute episodes of schizophrenia, increased norepinephrine levels have been associated with increases in positive and negative symptoms, and, in chronic schizophrenia, decreased norepinephrine levels have been associated with increased negative symptoms (van Kammen and Kelley 1991; van Kammen et al. 1990). These considerations provide the empirical basis for the use of noradrenergic agents to treat negative symptoms.

Three studies have examined the effect of propranolol, a β_1- and β_2-blocker, on negative symptomatology. Two of the studies examined the comparative efficacy of propranolol versus neuroleptics. Peet et al. (1981) found that propranolol had no beneficial effect and may actually worsen negative symptoms. In contrast, Eccleston et al. (1985) reported that propranolol significantly reduced the level of negative symptoms; however, reductions in negative symptoms coincided with reductions in positive symptoms. Pugh et al. (1983) examined the efficacy of propranolol as an adjunct to continued neuroleptic treatment. These investigators found that propranolol had no significant effect on either BPRS total or anergia factor scores.

One study examined the effect of clonidine, an α_2 presynaptic receptor agonist, on negative symptoms. van Kammen et al. (1989) found that negative symptoms decreased in 4 of 13 patients, but the decrease was associated with a decrease in positive symptoms as well.

Maprotiline and imipramine are noradrenergic reuptake blockers used to treat depression. Yamagami and Soejima (1989) reported that maprotiline, when given as an adjunct to neuroleptics, resulted in a greater than 50% decrease in negative symptoms. The authors did not provide information about the effect of maprotiline on positive or depressive symptoms. Siris and colleagues (1991) found that imipramine had a significant effect on negative symptoms in a group of patients with schizophrenia defined by the presence of a postpsychotic depression. The reduction in negative symptoms was not associated with a reduction in psychotic symptoms; data on concurrent changes in depressive symptoms and EPS were not provided.

Summary. Relatively few studies have examined the effect of noradrenergic agents on negative symptoms. The majority of studies have found these agents to be effective for reducing negative symptoms, but they are characterized by the same methodological limitations as the dopamine agonist studies.

Serotonergic Agents

Complex interactions occur between serotonergic and dopaminergic neuronal systems (Bleich et al. 1988). Serotonin (5-HT) containing neurons originating from the medial and dorsal raphe nuclei have axoaxonal synaptic connections with dopamine circuits. 5-HT appears to have an inhibitory modulatory effect on dopamine function via 5-HT receptors at the dopamine terminals. Clozapine's 5-HT_2 antagonism and its purported efficacy in the treatment of negative symptoms (see "Clozapine" subsection below) have also stimulated interest in the use of serotonergic agents for the treatment of negative symptoms. Both 5-HT antagonists and agonists have been used to treat negative symptoms.

Four studies have evaluated the efficacy of fenfluramine—an agent that blocks 5-HT reuptake and depletes intracellular 5-HT—for the treatment of negative symptoms. Stahl et al. (1985) reported that fenfluramine decreased negative symptoms in three of eight patients. However, two of the three patients who had a reduction in negative symptoms also exhibited marked improvements in positive symptoms. Alphs et al. (1989) found that high-dose (180 mg/day), but not low-dose, fenfluramine was associated with a significant reduction in negative symptoms. In contrast, two studies could not document a beneficial effect for fenfluramine (Marshall et al. 1989; Shore et al. 1985). It is interesting that in the study by Stahl and associates (1985), the three patients who experienced negative symptom improvement were receiving high-dose fenfluramine (≥ 180 mg/day), and in the two studies that failed to find a beneficial effect (Marshall et al. 1989; Shore et al. 1985), the maximum fenfluramine dosages were below the dosage observed to be effective in the study by Alphs et al. (1989).

Two studies used selective 5-HT reuptake inhibitors to treat negative symptoms (Goff et al. 1990; Silver and Nassar 1992). In an open trial, adjunctive fluoxetine was found to decrease negative, positive, and depressive symptoms significantly (Goff et al. 1990), and in a double-blind study, adjunctive fluvoxamine, compared with placebo, produced a significantly greater decrease in negative symptoms (Silver and Nassar 1992). Fluvoxamine treatment was also associated with significant decreases in positive and depressive symptoms and EPS.

Two placebo-controlled, double-blind studies examined the efficacy of ritanserin—a 5-HT_{1c} and 5-HT_2 antagonist—for negative symptoms (Duinkerke et al. 1993; Reyntjens et al. 1986). Both studies used ritanserin as an adjunctive treatment to stable neuroleptic treatment, and both studies selected patients with prominent negative symptomatology. Reyntjens et al. reported that ritanserin produced significant reductions in the BPRS anergia factor. This reduction in negative symptoms occurred concurrently with reductions in the BPRS total score and in EPS. Duinkerke et al. also found ritanserin to be effective for negative symptoms. In addition to the significant reduction in SANS total score, they observed that ritanserin treatment resulted in a significant reduction in the BPRS depressive mood item and a trend reduction in the BPRS total score. Reduction in BPRS total score was significantly correlated with reduction in SANS total score. The results of these studies are consistent with a role for 5-HT antagonists in the treatment of negative symptoms but are not conclusive because the response of primary versus secondary negative symptoms was not differentiated. The results are also consistent with the hypothesis that antipsychotics with potent serotonergic antagonistic actions (e.g., clozapine and risperidone; see "Atypical Antipsychotics" section below) may be particularly effective for negative symptoms.

Finally, amitriptyline and mianserin, antidepressants with combined serotonergic and noradrenergic activities, have been used for the treatment of negative symptoms. Prusoff et al. (1979) conducted a double-blind study and found that when amitriptyline was added to neuroleptics, it had no beneficial effect on the BPRS anergia factor scores. Mizuki et al. (1992) found that mianserin decreased BPRS anergia factor scores when given in an open trial. The reduction in BPRS anergia factor scores occurred independently of changes in positive or depressive symptoms but concurrently with changes in anxiety symptoms.

Summary. Most studies have found that serotonergic agents are effective for reducing negative symptoms. The studies of 5-HT_2 antagonists are potentially of interest, but adequate attempts have not been made to control for potential confounding variables (i.e., concurrent change in positive and depressive symptoms).

Anticholinergics

Tandon and Greden (1989) have argued that cholinergic hyperactivity may be related to the production of negative symptoms. This may be either a direct effect of cholinergic activity or an indirect effect through the cholinergic system's interaction with dopaminergic pathways. A cholinergic hypothesis of negative symptoms is supported by neuroanatomical observations. Specifically, the basal ganglia and neocortex, brain regions that have been implicated in the neuroanatomy of negative symptoms, receive cholinergic input (Robinson 1985). There is considerable evidence for reciprocal interactions between dopaminergic and cholinergic pathways in these areas (Beani and Bianchi 1973; Costall and Naylor 1972; Pepeu and Bartolini 1968). If cholinergic hyperactivity is related to negative symptomatology, then anticholinergics could be a potential treatment for these symptoms.

In a series of case reports, adjunctive anticholinergic treatment was found to increase energy, elevate mood, and increase socialization in patients with chronic schizophrenia (Fisch 1987; Jellinek 1977). Tandon et al. (1988) reported that four of five patients who participated in an open trial of trihexyphenidyl exhibited decreased negative symptomatology, with the change in negative symptoms occurring independently of positive symptoms or EPS.

Five double-blind studies have examined the effects of anticholinergic treatment on negative symptoms. M. M. Singh and Kay (1979) reported that anticholinergics reversed the effect of neuroleptic treatment, with both positive and negative symptoms worsening. In a later study, they found that adjunctive anticholinergics worsened positive symptoms but did not affect negative symptoms (M. M. Singh et al. 1987). Tandon and colleagues (1990, 1992) demonstrated that brief (2 days) biperiden treatment in neuroleptic-free patients with schizophrenia exacerbates positive symptoms and decreases the level of negative symptoms. Finally, Goff et al. (1994) examined the efficacy of trihexyphenidyl in drug-free patients with schizophrenia. They found that there were no significant differences in efficacy between trihexyphenidyl and placebo for negative symptoms.

Summary. Although open-label studies have suggested a beneficial therapeutic effect of anticholinergics for negative symptoms, the results of double-blind treatment studies have not demonstrated a beneficial effect of these agents for negative symptoms. In addition, two studies found that anticholinergic agents may be associated with an increased risk of psychotic symptom exacerbation regardless of the patient's neuroleptic status. The failure of double-blind treatment studies to demonstrate a beneficial effect of anticholinergic treatment precludes recommending these agents for treatment of negative symptoms.

Atypical Antipsychotics

The negative symptom efficacy of three atypical antipsychotics—clozapine, risperidone, and remoxipride—has been examined extensively. These agents differ from traditional neuroleptics in their pharmacological properties, mechanisms of action, and side-effect profiles. These differences, discussed below, provide the basis for hypotheses of their possible enhanced efficacy for the treatment of negative symptoms.

Clozapine

Clozapine was originally developed in 1960 but was not approved for use in the United States until 1990 (Baldessarini and Frankenburg 1991). Clozapine acts at a number of neurotransmitter receptors (Baldessarini and Frankenburg 1991); it has relatively low affinity for the dopamine D_1 and D_2 receptors (with relatively greater activity at D_1) as well as for the noradrenergic α_2 receptor. Clozapine has high affinity for the dopamine D_4, the serotonin 5-HT_2, the muscarinic M_1, the noradrenergic α_1, and the histamine receptors. Clozapine is associated with a low incidence of EPS, which may be related to either its low affinity for D_2 receptors or its relatively high 5-HT_2/D_2 affinity ratio.

Several studies have examined the efficacy of clozapine for negative symptoms. The largest of these studies was the multicenter controlled study by Kane and colleagues (1988). They examined the comparative efficacy of clozapine versus chlorpromazine in treatment-resistant inpatients with schizophrenia and found that clozapine was significantly more effective than chlorpromazine in reducing BPRS anergia factor scores. They also found that clozapine significantly reduced the levels of positive symptoms and EPS. Similar results were reported by Pickar et al. (1992). They found that clozapine treatment of inpatients with schizophrenia was associated with significant reductions in the BPRS anergia factor score, positive symptoms, and EPS. However, when negative symptoms were directly assessed with the SANS, these investigators did not find clozapine treatment to have a significant effect. Breier et al. (1994) conducted a study of partially responsive outpatients with schizophrenia and reported a significant difference between clozapine and haloperidol for SANS total negative symptoms. The difference was due to nonsignificant increases in negative symptoms in the haloperidol-treated patients and nonsignificant decreases in negative symptoms in the clozapine-treated patients. There was also concurrent improvement in positive symptoms but not EPS. To specifically examine the effect of clozapine on primary negative symptoms, Breier and colleagues dichotomized the patients into deficit (characterized by the presence of primary and enduring negative symptoms) and nondeficit (characterized by the absence of primary and enduring negative symptoms) subgroups and observed the change in negative symptoms in response to clozapine treatment in both subgroups. There was no change in the mean level of negative symptoms in the clozapine-treated deficit patients, and none of the deficit patients met criteria for clinically significant reduction in negative symptoms. In contrast, there were nonsignificant reductions in the mean level of negative symptoms in the clozapine-treated nondeficit patients, and 3 of 10 nondeficit patients exhibited a greater than 20% reduction in negative symptoms.

The apparent differences in negative symptom responsiveness among these studies may be related to the following factors:

- Kane et al. (1988) and Pickar et al. (1992) documented clozapine's effect on negative symptoms with the BPRS anergia factor, whereas neither Pickar et al. nor Breier et al. (1994) found clozapine to be an effective treatment for negative symptoms as assessed by the SANS. The BPRS anergia factor is a proxy measure for negative symptoms and includes items that may be sensitive to the effect of EPS (e.g., psychomotor retardation). Alternatively, but less likely, the SANS may not be sensitive enough to detect pharmacologically related changes in negative symptoms.
- The Kane et al. and Pickar et al. studies were conducted with inpatients, who entered the studies with high levels of EPS. These patients experienced significant reductions in the level of EPS, reductions that occurred concurrently with the significant reduction in the BPRS anergia factor scores. In contrast, the Breier et al. study was conducted with outpatients. The patients entered the study with low levels of EPS, and no significant reductions in these symptoms occurred with clozapine treatment.

Risperidone

Risperidone is a very potent 5-HT_2 and D_2 antagonist. Risperidone has been shown to be at least as effective as traditional neuroleptics for the treatment of positive symptoms (Chouinard et al. 1993; Wilms et al. 1992). It has also been shown, within certain dosage ranges, to be less likely than haloperidol to cause EPS (Chouinard et al. 1993).

The efficacy of risperidone for negative symptoms has been examined in open-label trials (Bersani et al. 1990; Mesotten et al. 1989; Roose et al. 1988), a single-blind study (Meco et al. 1989), and double-blind studies (Borison et al. 1992; Claus et al. 1992; Chouinard et al. 1993; Marder and Meibach 1994; Wilms et al. 1992). Roose et al. (1988) reported that risperidone increased sociability and decreased positive symptoms and EPS. Mesotten et al. (1989) found that risperidone, in dosages up to 20 mg/day, decreased BPRS anergia factor scores and positive and depressive symptoms. Higher dosages were associated with increased sedation and a loss of the beneficial effect on the BPRS anergia factor. Bersani et al. (1990) reported, in patients who met criteria for predominant negative symptoms and poor response to traditional neuroleptics, that risperidone treatment resulted in a significant decrease in negative symptoms as assessed with either the BPRS anergia factor or the SANS, as well as significant improvements in hallucinations and delusions. Meco et al. (1989) compared risperidone with placebo in a single-blind crossover study and found that risperidone treatment was associated with a significant improvement in positive, negative, depressive, and anxiety symptoms.

The results of the double-blind studies are less encouraging with respect to risperidone's effect on negative symptoms. Borison et al. (1992) did not find a differential effect of risperidone versus either haloperidol or placebo for negative symptoms. Claus et al. (1992) found no significant differences between risperidone and haloperidol efficacy for negative symptoms, although a greater proportion of risperidone-treated patients exhibited reductions in negative symptoms. Wilms et al. (1992) also did not find any significant differences between risperidone and haloperidol efficacy. In the United States–Canadian multicenter study (Chouinard et al. 1993; Marder and Meibach 1994), multiple risperidone doses were compared with a single haloperidol dose. In the 6 Canadian centers, Chouinard et al. (1993) reported that risperidone, 6 mg/day, produced a significantly greater reduction in negative symptoms than placebo and produced, at a trend level, a greater reduction in negative symptoms than haloperidol. This risperidone dose also produced a significant reduction, compared with placebo, in positive symptoms. In the 20 United States centers (Marder and Meibach 1994), risperidone, both 6 mg/day and 16 mg/day, but not haloperidol, produced significantly greater reductions in negative symptoms than placebo. Both risperidone doses also produced greater reductions in positive symptoms than placebo. There were no significant differences between risperidone and haloperidol for negative symptoms.

Remoxipride

Remoxipride is a specific D_2-receptor antagonist, with preferential affinity for extrastriatal D_2 receptors (Wadworth and Heel 1990). It has little affinity for serotonergic, muscarinic, α_1 noradrenergic, or histamine receptors (Wadworth and Heel 1990). Remoxipride has been found to be an effective antipsychotic, and most important, it is associated with low levels of EPS (Wadworth and Heel 1990). (Remoxipride treatment has been found to be associated with the development of aplastic anemia and is currently not in development in the United States.)

Four open trials have examined the effect of remoxipride on negative symptoms (Chouinard 1987; den Boer et al. 1986; Laursen and Gerlach 1986; Lindstrom et al. 1985). Three studies reported that remoxipride treatment resulted in reductions in BPRS measures of positive symptoms and the BPRS anergia factor (den Boer et al. 1986; Laursen and Gerlach 1986; Lindstrom et al. 1985). In contrast, Chouinard (1987) found no differential effect for remoxipride on the BPRS anergia factor, when compared with BPRS ratings performed while patients were on haloperidol.

There have been nine multicenter double-blind comparisons of remoxipride versus haloperidol (Ahlfors et al. 1990; Andersen et al. 1990; den Boer et al. 1990; Deo et al. 1990; Lapierre et al. 1990; Laux et al. 1990; Lindstrom et al. 1990; Mendlewicz et al. 1990; Patris et al. 1990) and one multicenter double-blind comparison of remoxipride versus chlorpromazine (Chouinard 1990). Six studies reported no difference between remoxipride and haloperidol for positive or negative symptoms (Ahlfors et al. 1990; Andersen et al. 1990; den Boer et al. 1990; Deo et al. 1990; Lindstrom et al. 1990; Mendlewicz et al. 1990). Laux et al. (1990) observed that remoxipride administered twice daily was more effective than either remoxipride administered thrice daily or haloperidol for negative symptoms. Patris et al. (1990) found that remoxipride was more effective than haloperidol for negative symptoms, but haloperidol was more effective than remoxipride for positive symptoms. Chouinard (1990) reported that remoxipride was significantly less effective than chlorpromazine for negative symptoms. Lapierre et al. (1990) did not provide enough information to draw any conclusions on the relative merits of remoxipride versus haloperidol.

Summary. The results of these studies suggest that clozapine is more effective, and risperidone and remoxipride may be more effective, than traditional neuroleptics for the treatment of secondary negative symptoms. Only one study has examined the effect of these agents on primary negative symptoms (Breier et al. 1994), and that study did not document a therapeutic effect of clozapine for these symptoms.

Conclusion

A broad range of effective treatments is available for secondary negative symptoms, which underscores the importance of the differential diagnosis for negative symptoms. However, despite more than 20 years of negative symptom treatment research, no proven pharmacological treatments are available for primary negative symptoms. The data, to date, are most supportive of the potential efficacy of dopamine agonists. Norepinephrine and 5-HT reuptake blockers may be useful for the treatment of primary negative symptoms; few data, to date, support the use of anti-7cholinergics in the treatment of primary negative symptoms. Atypical antipsychotics have been shown to be effective for the treatment of negative symptoms, but scant attention has been paid to whether their negative symptom efficacy is restricted to secondary negative symptoms.

The development of effective treatments for primary negative symptoms remains one of the most challenging tasks confronting clinicians treating patients with schizophrenia.

References

Adan F, Siris SG: Trials of adjunctive alprazolam in "negative symptom" patients. Can J Psychiatry 34:326–328, 1989

Ahlfors UG, Rimon R, Appelberg B, et al: Remoxipride and haloperidol in schizophrenia: a double-blind multicentre study. Acta Psychiatr Scand 82:99–103, 1990

Alpert M, Friedhoff AJ, Marcos LR, et al: Paradoxical reaction to L-dopa in schizophrenic patients. Am J Psychiatry 135:1329–1332, 1978

Alphs LD, Lafferman JA, Ross L, et al: Fenfluramine treatment of negative symptoms in older schizophrenic inpatients. Psychopharmacol Bull 25:149–153, 1989

Andersen J, Korner A, Ostergaard P, et al: A double-blind comparative multicentre study of remoxipride and haloperidol in schizophrenia. Acta Psychiatr Scand 82:104–107, 1990

Andreasen NC: The Scale for Assessment of Negative Symptoms (SANS). Iowa City, IA, University of Iowa, 1981

Andreasen NC, Olsen SA: Negative vs. positive schizophrenia: definition and validation. Arch Gen Psychiatry 39:297–302, 1982

Angrist B, Sathananthan G, Gershon S: Behavioral effects of L-dopa in schizophrenic patients. Psychopharmacology (Berl) 31:1–12, 1973

Angrist B, Rotrosen J, Gershon S: Differential effects of amphetamine and neuroleptics on negative vs. positive symptoms in schizophrenia. Psychopharmacology (Berl) 72:17–19, 1980

Angrist B, Peselow E, Rubinstein M, et al: Partial improvement in negative schizophrenic symptoms after amphetamine. Psychopharmacology (Berl) 78:128–130, 1982

Baldessarini RJ, Frankenburg FR: Clozapine: a novel antipsychotic agent. N Engl J Med 324:746–754, 1991

Beani L, Bianchi C: Effect of amantadine on cerebral acetylcholine release and content in the guinea pig. Neuropharmacology 12:283–289, 1973

Berrios GE: Positive and negative symptoms and Jackson: a conceptual history. Arch Gen Psychiatry 42:95–97, 1985

Bersani G, Bressa GM, Meco G, et al: Combined serotonin-5HT$_2$ and dopamine-D$_2$ antagonism in schizophrenia: clinical, extrapyramidal and neuroendocrine response in a preliminary study with risperidone (R 64 766). Human Psychopharmacology 5:225–231, 1990

Bleich A, Brown S-L, Kahn R, et al: The role of serotonin in schizophrenia. Schizophr Bull 14:297–315, 1988

Borison RL, Pathiraja AP, Diamond BI: Risperidone: clinical safety and efficacy in schizophrenia. Psychopharmacol Bull 28:213–218, 1992

Breier A, Buchanan RW, Kirkpatrick B, et al: Effects of clozapine on positive and negative symptoms in outpatients with schizophrenia. Am J Psychiatry 151:20–26, 1994

Bruno A, Bruno SC: Effects of L-dopa on pharmacological parkinsonism. Acta Psychiatr Scand 42:264–271, 1966

Bucci L: The negative symptoms of schizophrenia and the monoamine oxidase inhibitors. Psychopharmacology (Berl) 91:104–108, 1987

Buchanan FH, Parton RV, Warren JW, et al: Double blind trial of L-dopa in chronic schizophrenia. Aust N Z J Psychiatry 9:269–271, 1975

Buchanan RW, Carpenter WT: Domains of psychopathology: concept and validity. J Nerv Ment Dis 182:193–204, 1994

Carpenter WT Jr, Buchanan RW: Domains of psychopathology relevant to the study of etiology and treatment of schizophrenia, in Schizophrenia: Scientific Progress. Edited by Schulz SC, Tamminga CT. New York, Oxford University Press, 1989, pp 13–22

Carpenter WT Jr, Conley RR: Therapeutic approaches to negative symptoms, in Negative Schizophrenic Symptoms: Pathophysiology and Clinical Implications. Edited by Greden JF, Tandon R. Washington, DC, American Psychiatric Press, 1991, pp 205–214

Carpenter WT Jr, Heinrichs DW, Alphs LD: Treatment of negative symptoms. Schizophr Bull 11:440–452, 1985

Carpenter WT Jr, Heinrichs DW, Wagman AMI: Deficit and non-deficit forms of schizophrenia: the concept. Am J Psychiatry 145:578–583, 1988

Cesarec Z, Nyman AK: Differential response to amphetamine in schizophrenia. Acta Psychiatr Scand 71:523–538, 1985

Chouinard G: Early phase II clinical trial of remoxipride in treatment of schizophrenia with measurements of prolactin and neuroleptic activity. J Clin Psychopharmacol 3:159–164, 1987

Chouinard G: A placebo-controlled clinical trial of remoxipride and chlorpromazine in newly admitted schizophrenic patients with acute exacerbation. Acta Psychiatr Scand 82:111–119, 1990

Chouinard G, Jones B, Remington G, et al: A Canadian multicenter placebo-controlled study of fixed doses of risperidone and haloperidol in the treatment of chronic schizophrenic patients. J Clin Psychopharmacol 13:25–40, 1993

Claus A, Bollen J, De Cuyper H, et al: Risperidone versus haloperidol in the treatment of chronic schizophrenic inpatients: a multicentre double-blind comparative study. Acta Psychiatr Scand 85:295–305, 1992

Costall B, Naylor RJ: Modification of amphetamine effects by intracerebrally administered anticholinergic agents. Life Sci 11:239–253, 1972

Crow TJ: The two-syndrome concept: origins and current status. Schizophr Bull 11:471–486, 1985

Csernansky JG, Lombrozo L, Gulevich GD, et al: Treatment of negative schizophrenic symptoms with alprazolam: a preliminary open-label study. J Clin Psychopharmacol 4:349–352, 1984

Csernansky JG, Riney SJ, Lombrozo L, et al: Double-blind comparison of alprazolam, diazepam, and placebo for the treatment of negative schizophrenic symptoms. Arch Gen Psychiatry 45:655–659, 1988

Davis KL, Kahn RS, Ko G, et al: Dopamine in schizophrenia: a review and reconceptualization. Am J Psychiatry 148:1474–1486, 1991

den Boer JA, Verhoeven WMA, Westenberg HGM: Remoxipride in schizophrenia: a preliminary report. Acta Psychiatr Scand 74:409–414, 1986 den Boer JA, Ravelli DP, Huisman J, et al: A double-blind comparative study of remoxipride and haloperidol in acute schizophrenia. Acta Psychiatr Scand 82:108–110, 1990

Deo R, Soni S, Rastogi SC, et al: Remoxipride and haloperidol in the acute phase of schizophrenia: a double-blind comparison. Acta Psychiatr Scand 82:120–124, 1990

Douyon R, Angrist B, Peselow E, et al: Neuroleptic augmentation with alprazolam: clinical effects and pharmacokinetic correlates. Am J Psychiatry 146:231–234, 1989

Duinkerke SJ, Botter PA, Jansen AAI, et al: Ritanserin, a selective 5-$HT_{2/1C}$ antagonist, and negative symptoms in schizophrenia: a placebo-controlled double-blind trial. Br J Psychiatry 163:451–455, 1993

Eccleston D, Fairbairn AF, Hassanyeh F, et al: The effect of propranolol and thioridazine on positive and negative symptoms of schizophrenia. Br J Psychiatry 147:623–630, 1985

Fisch RZ: Trihexyphenidyl abuse: therapeutic implications for negative symptoms of schizophrenia? Acta Psychiatr Scand 75:91–94, 1987

Gattaz WF, Rost W, Hubner CvK, et al: Acute and subchronic effects of low-dose bromocriptine in haloperidol-treated schizophrenics. Biol Psychiatry 25:247–255, 1989

Gerbaldo H, Demisch L, Lehmann C-O, et al: The effect of OPC-4392, a partial dopamine receptor agonist on negative symptoms: results of an open study. Pharmacopsychiatry 21:387–388, 1988

Gerlach J, Luhdorf K: The effect of L-dopa on young patients with simple schizophrenia, treated with neuroleptic drugs. Psychopharmacology (Berl) 44:105–109, 1975

Goff DC, Brotman AW, Waites M, et al: Trial of fluoxetine added to neuroleptics for treatment-resistant schizophrenic patients. Am J Psychiatry 147:492–494, 1990

Goff DC, Amico E, Dreyfuss D, et al: A placebo-controlled trial of trihexyphenidyl in unmedicated patients with schizophrenia. Am J Psychiatry 151:429–431, 1994

Goldberg E: Akinesia, tardive dysmentia, and frontal lobe disorder in schizophrenia. Schizophr Bull 11:255–263, 1985

Goldberg SC: Negative and deficit symptoms in schizophrenia do respond to neuroleptics. Schizophr Bull 11:453–456, 1985

Herrera JM, Alvarez WA, Freinhar JP, et al: Adjunctive clonazepam in the treatment of chronic schizophrenia. Int J Psychosom 38:17–20, 1991

Jellinek T: Mood elevating effect of trihexyphenidyl and biperiden in individuals taking antipsychotic medication. Diseases of the Nervous System 38:353–355, 1977

Kane J, Honigfeld G, Singer J, et al: Clozapine for the treatment-resistant schizophrenic: a double-blind comparison with chlorpromazine. Arch Gen Psychiatry 45:789–796, 1988

Kay SR, Opler LA: L-dopa in the treatment of negative schizophrenic symptoms: a single-subject experimental study. Int J Psychiatry Med 15:293–298, 1985–1986

King DJ: Dopamine agonists for negative symptoms in schizophrenia. Br J Clin Pharmacol 6:541–542, 1978

Kraepelin E: Dementia Præcox and Paraphrenia. Translated by Barclay RM. Edited by Robertson GM. Edinburgh, E & S Livingstone, 1919

Lapierre YD, Nair NPV, Chouinard G, et al: A controlled dose-ranging study of remoxipride and haloperidol in schizophrenia—a Canadian multicentre trial. Acta Psychiatr Scand 82:72–76, 1990

Laursen AL, Gerlach J: Antipsychotic effect of remoxipride, a new substituted benzamide with selective antidopaminergic activity. Acta Psychiatr Scand 73:17–21, 1986

Laux G, Klieser E, Schroder HG, et al: A double-blind multicentre study comparing remoxipride, two and three times daily, with haloperidol in schizophrenia. Acta Psychiatr Scand 82:125–129, 1990

Levi-Minzi S, Bermanzohn PC, Siris SG: Bromocriptine for "negative" schizophrenia. Compr Psychiatry 32:210–216, 1991

Lindstrom L, Besev G, Stening G, et al: An open study of remoxipride, a benzamide derivative, in schizophrenia. Psychopharmacology (Berl) 86:241–243, 1985

Lindstrom LH, Wieselgren I-M, Struwe G, et al: A double-blind comparative multicentre study of remoxipride and haloperidol in schizophrenia. Acta Psychiatr Scand 82:130–135, 1990

Lingjaerde O, Engstrand E, Ellingsen P, et al: Antipsychotic effect of diazepam when given in addition to neuroleptics in chronic psychotic patients: a double-blind clinical trial. Current Therapeutic Research 26:505–514, 1979

Marder SR, Meibach RC: Risperidone in the treatment of schizophrenia. Am J Psychiatry 151:825–835, 1994

Marshall BD, Glynn SM, Midha KK, et al: Adverse effects of fenfluramine in treatment refractory schizophrenia. J Clin Psychopharmacol 9:110–115, 1989

Meco G, Bedini L, Bonifati V, et al: Risperidone in the treatment of chronic schizophrenia with tardive dyskinesia. Current Therapeutic Research 46:876–883, 1989

Mendlewicz J, de Bleeker E, Cosyns P, et al: A double-blind comparative study of remoxipride and haloperidol in schizophrenic and schizophreniform disorders. Acta Psychiatr Scand 82:138–141, 1990

Mesotten F, Suy E, Pietquin M, et al: Therapeutic effect and safety of increasing doses of risperidone (R 64 766) in psychotic patients. Psychopharmacology (Berl) 99:445–449, 1989

Mizuki Y, Kajimura N, Kai S, et al: Effects of mianserin in chronic schizophrenia. Prog Neuropsychopharmacol Biol Psychiatry 16:517–528, 1992

Nestoros JN, Suranyi-Cadotte BE, Spees RC, et al: Diazepam in high doses is effective in schizophrenia. Prog Neuropsychopharmacol Biol Psychiatry 6:513–516, 1982

Nestoros JN, Nair NPV, Pulman JR, et al: High doses of diazepam improve neuroleptic-resistant chronic schizophrenic patients. Psychopharmacology (Berl) 81:42–47, 1983

Ogura C, Kishimoto A, Nakao T: Clinical effects of L-dopa on schizophrenia. Current Therapeutic Research 20:308–318, 1976

Olbrich R, Schanz H: The effect of the partial dopamine agonist terguride on negative symptoms in schizophrenia. Pharmacopsychiatry 21:389–390, 1988

Olbrich R, Schanz H: An evaluation of the partial dopamine agonist terguride regarding positive symptoms reduction in schizophrenia. J Neural Transm Gen Sect 84:233–236, 1991

Overall JE, Gorham DE: The Brief Psychiatric Rating Scale. Psychol Rep 10:799–812, 1962

Patris M, Agussol P, Alby JM, et al: A double-blind multicentre comparison of remoxipride, at two dose levels, and haloperidol. Acta Psychiatr Scand 82:78–82, 1990

Peet M, Bethell MS, Coates A, et al: Propranolol in schizophrenia, I: comparison of propranolol, chlorpromazine and placebo. Br J Psychiatry 139:105–111, 1981

Pepeu G, Bartolini A: Effect of psychoactive drugs on the output of acetylcholine from the cerebral cortex of the cat. Eur J Pharmacol 4:254–263, 1968

Perenyi A, Goswami U, Freccska E, et al: L-deprenyl in treating negative symptoms of schizophrenia (letter). Psychiatry Res 42:189–191, 1992

Pickar D, Owen RR, Litman RE, et al: Clinical and biologic response to clozapine in patients with schizophrenia: crossover comparison with fluphenazine. Arch Gen Psychiatry 49:345–353, 1992

Prusoff BA, Williams DH, Weissman MM, et al: Treatment of secondary depression in schizophrenia. Arch Gen Psychiatry 36:569–575, 1979

Pugh CR, Steinert J, Priest RG: Propranolol in schizophrenia: a double blind, placebo controlled trial of propranolol as an adjunct to neuroleptic medication. Br J Psychiatry 143:151–155, 1983

Reyntjens A, Gelders YG, Hoppenbrouwers M-L JA, et al: Thymosthenic effects of ritanserin (R 55667), a centrally acting serotonin-S_2 receptor blocker. Drug Development Research 8:205–211, 1986

Robinson SE: Cholinergic pathways in the brain, in Central Cholinergic Mechanisms and Adaptive Dysfunctions. Edited by Singh MM, Warburton DM, Lal H. New York, Plenum, 1985, pp 37–61

Roose K, Gelders Y, Heylen S: Risperidone (R 64 766) in psychotic patients: a first clinical therapeutic exploration. Acta Psychiatr Belg 88:233–241, 1988

Seibyl J, Krystal J, Johnson R, et al: Mazindol augmentation of typical antipsychotics in negative symptom schizophrenics (Abstract 148.6). Society for Neuroscience Abstracts 17:354, 1991

Seibyl J, Erdos J, Karper L, et al: Long-term mazindol augmentation of neuroleptic in negative schizophrenia (Abstract 95.4). Society for Neuroscience Abstracts 18:202, 1992

Shore D, Korpi ER, Bigelow LB, et al: Fenfluramine and chronic schizophrenia. Biol Psychiatry 20:329–352, 1985

Silver H, Nassar A: Fluvoxamine improves negative symptoms in treated chronic schizophrenia: an add-on double-blind, placebo-controlled study. Biol Psychiatry 31:698–704, 1992

Singh AN, Saxena B, Nelson HL: A controlled clinical study of trazodone in chronic schizophrenic patients with pronounced depressive symptomatology. Current Therapeutic Research 23:485–501, 1978

Singh MM, Kay SR: Therapeutic antagonism between anticholinergic antiparkinsonism agents and neuroleptics in schizophrenia. Neuropsychobiology 5:74–86, 1979

Singh MM, Kay SR, Opler LA: Anticholinergic-neuroleptic antagonism in terms of positive and negative symptoms of schizophrenia: implications for psychobiological subtyping. Psychol Med 17:38–48, 1987

Siris SG, Morgan V, Fagerstrom R, et al: Adjunctive imipramine in the treatment of post-psychotic depression: a controlled trial. Arch Gen Psychiatry 44:533–539, 1987

Siris SG, Bermanzohn PC, Gonzalez A, et al: The use of antidepressants for negative symptoms in a subset of schizophrenic patients. Psychopharmacol Bull 27:331–335, 1991

Stahl SM, Uhr SB, Berger PA: Pilot study on the effects of fenfluramine on negative symptoms in twelve schizophrenic inpatients. Biol Psychiatry 20:1098–1102, 1985

Strauss JS, Carpenter WT, Bartko JJ: The diagnosis and understanding of schizophrenia, part 3: speculations on the processes that underlie schizophrenic symptoms and signs. Schizophr Bull 11:61–75, 1974

Tandon R, Greden JF: Cholinergic hyperactivity and negative schizophrenic symptoms. Arch Gen Psychiatry 46:745–753, 1989

Tandon R, Greden JF, Silk KR: Treatment of negative schizophrenic symptoms with trihexyphenidyl. J Clin Psychopharmacol 8:212–215, 1988

Tandon R, Mann NA, Eisner WH, et al: Effect of anticholinergic medication on positive and negative symptoms in medication-free schizophrenic patients. Psychiatry Res 31:235–241, 1990

Tandon R, DeQuardo JR, Goodson J, et al: Effect of anticholinergics on positive and negative symptoms in schizophrenia. Psychopharmacol Bull 28:297–302, 1992

Tassin JP: NE/DA interactions in prefrontal cortex and their possible roles as neuromodulators in schizophrenia. J Neural Transm Gen Sect 36:135–162, 1992

van Kammen DP, Boronow JJ: Dextro-amphetamine diminishes negative symptoms in schizophrenia. Int Clin Psychopharmacol 3:111–121, 1988

van Kammen DP, Kelley M: Dopamine and norepinephrine activity in schizophrenia: an integrative perspective. Schizophr Res 4:173–191, 1991

van Kammen DP, Peters JL, van Kammen WB, et al: Clonidine treatment of schizophrenia: can we predict treatment response? Psychiatry Res 27:297–311, 1989

van Kammen DP, Peters J, Yao J, et al: Norepinephrine in acute exacerbations of chronic schizophrenia. Arch Gen Psychiatry 47:161–168, 1990

Wadworth AN, Heel RC: Remoxipride: a review of its pharmacodynamic and pharmacokinetic properties, and therapeutic potential in schizophrenia. Drugs 40:863–879, 1990

Weinberger DR: Implications of normal brain development for the pathogenesis of schizophrenia. Arch Gen Psychiatry 44:660–669, 1987

Wilms G, Van Ongeval C, Baert AL, et al: Ventricular enlargement, clinical correlates and treatment outcome in chronic schizophrenic inpatients. Acta Psychiatr Scand 85:306–312, 1992

Wing JK, Brown GW: Institutionalism and Schizophrenia: A Comparative Study of Three Mental Hospitals 1960–1968. Cambridge, MA, Cambridge University Press, 1970

Wolf M-A, Diener J-M, Lajeunesse C, et al: Low-dose bromocriptine in neuroleptic-resistant schizophrenia: a pilot study. Biol Psychiatry 31:1166–1168, 1992

Wolkowitz OM, Pickar D, Doran AR, et al: Combination alprazolam-neuroleptic treatment of the positive and negative symptoms of schizophrenia. Am J Psychiatry 143:85–87, 1986

Wolkowitz OM, Breier A, Doran A, et al: Alprazolam augmentation of the antipsychotic effects of fluphenazine in schizophrenic patients: preliminary results. Arch Gen Psychiatry 45:664–671, 1988

Yamagami S, Soejima K: Effect of maprotiline combined with conventional neuroleptics against negative symptoms of chronic schizophrenia. Drugs Exp Clin Res 15:171–176, 1989

CHAPTER 10

Treatment of Depression in Patients With Schizophrenia

Samuel G. Siris, M.D.

Epidemiological evidence has demonstrated that a substantial proportion of patients with histories of psychosis diagnosed as meeting criteria for schizophrenia manifest prominent depression-like symptomatology subsequent to the partial or complete resolution of their psychoses (Barnes et al. 1989; Bartels and Drake 1988; Breier et al. 1991; Harrow et al. 1993; Hirsch et al. 1989; Johnson 1988; Siris 1991; Siris et al. 1981). The modal frequency of depression reported in these studies suggests that approximately 25% of patients develop depression, although the rate of reported occurrences varies considerably, presumably based on sample differences, length of observation, and the criteria used to indicate the presence of depression (McGlashan and Carpenter 1976; Siris 1991). Nevertheless, the diagnosis of depression is important for many reasons. The state of depression can contribute to patients' suffering and reduction in functional capability and may well predispose to mortality through suicide (Caldwell and Gottesman 1990; Roy 1986; Shuwall and Siris 1994). Indeed, the rate of suicide in patients with schizophrenia has been estimated to be as high as 10%. Furthermore, it is crucial to recognize the associated state of depression in schizophrenia because it is often treatable.

Differential Diagnosis

The proper treatment of the associated state of depression in the course of schizophrenia begins with a differential diagnosis. A phenocopy of depression can result from organic factors, neuroleptic-induced dysphoria, extrapyramidal side effects such as akinesia or akathisia, the so-called negative symptom state of schizophrenia, acute or chronic disappointment reactions, the prodrome of psychotic relapse, or the occurrence of schizoaffective disorder. Aside from these, depression may also occur during the course of schizophrenia in a form that is a component of the patient's underlying set of biological diatheses. The following paragraphs therefore attempt to differentiate these various clinical conditions, with an eye toward guiding appropriate treatment.

Organic Factors

Many medical conditions can predispose patients with schizophrenia to syndromes resembling depression (Bartels and Drake 1988, 1989). These include anemia, cancer, endocrine disorders, infectious diseases, and neurological conditions. It is obvious that in each of these situations, optimal therapy involves the assessment and treatment of the underlying medical conditions. In addition, a number of commonly prescribed medications can lead to the emergence of depressive symptomatology. These include a variety of antihypertension and cardiac medications such as β-blockers, sedative-hypnotics, sulfonamides, and indomethacin. Other medications can predispose patients to depression when they are discontinued (e.g., corticosteroids and psychostimulants). When patients with schizophrenia who appear depressed have been treated with any potentially depressogenic medications, appropriate treatment trials with alternative agents are indicated to determine whether a more favorable balance of treatment effects and side effects is possible.

The emergence of depressive-like symptomatology can also be caused by a variety of substances of abuse, either when they are used acutely or chronically or when they are discontinued. Commonly used and abused substances that often cause depressive effects are alcohol, cannabis, and cocaine. Patients who experience these effects should obviously discontinue these substances that predispose to depression. Stimulants may have to be discontinued gradually, however. Nicotine and caffeine are even more commonly self-administered; patients with schizophrenia frequently use these substances to excess, and when their use is reduced or discontinued, it can lead to dysphoric states that are easily confused with depression. In the case of tobacco smoking, replacement with a nicotine patch is possible, and in the case of caffeine, it should be recognized that some patients actually do best if they continue a moderate amount of intake of this agent as long as it does not contribute to their being nervous, physically jittery, or unable to sleep.

Neuroleptic-Induced Dysphoria

Controversy exists about whether neuroleptic agents can generate dysphoric states directly in patients. Although anecdotal reports suggest that this is possible, systematic investigations involving acute neuroleptic treatment of patients with schizophrenia often do not support this hypothesis (Knights and Hirsch 1981; Moller and von Zerssen 1986; Siris 1991). A theoretical basis exists for postulating the existence of neuroleptic-induced dysphoria because neuroleptic agents interfere with dopaminergic neurotransmission, and dopamine pathways are involved in central nervous system "reward" pathways (Harrow et al. 1993; Wise 1982). Thus, if the experience of reward or pleasure were reduced by a neuroleptic, the resultant state could be difficult to distinguish from the anhedonia of depression. Indeed, a number of early reports appeared to substantiate depression as a side effect of neuroleptic medication (DeAlarcon and Carney 1969; Floru et al. 1975; Galdi et al. 1981; Johnson 1981).

However, more recently, three lines of evidence have suggested that appropriately administered neuroleptic agents might not predispose to the emergence of depressive states. First, several studies that closely followed patients with schizophrenia through their course of neuroleptic treatment for acute episodes of psychosis tended to find a decrease in depressive symptomatology during treatment (Green et al. 1990; Hirsch et al. 1989; Knights and Hirsch 1981; Leff et al. 1988; Moller and von Zerssen 1982; Strian et al. 1982; Szymanski et al. 1983). A second group of studies found that patients with schizophrenia being treated with neuroleptics did not manifest more depressive symptoms than similar patients not being treated with neuroleptics (Hirsch et al. 1973, 1989; Hogarty and Munetz 1984; Wistedt and Palmstierna 1983). Finally, a third set of studies revealed that when depressed and nondepressed schizophrenic patient groups were compared, the depressed group was not found to be receiving higher neuroleptic doses or to have higher neuroleptic blood levels when these were measured (Bandelow et al. 1991; Barnes et al. 1989; Berrios and Bulbena 1987; Roy 1984; Roy et al. 1983; Siris et al. 1988b). Nevertheless, occasional well-designed studies still suggest that neuroleptics can play a role in the generation of depressive symptomatology (Harrow et al. 1993), and it is certainly possible that neuroleptics may be a factor in at least individual cases. Therefore, the widely respected strategy of minimal but continuous neuroleptic dosing in patients with schizophrenia is supported, especially for continuation and maintenance treatment (Carpenter et al. 1987; Herz et al. 1991; Hogarty et al. 1988; Jolley and Hirsch 1989; Kane et al. 1983; Marder et al. 1987).

Extrapyramidal Side Effects

Akinesia and akathisia are two side effects of neuroleptic medication that can clearly present with phenocopy symptoms of depression.

Neuroleptic-induced akinesia. Akinesia has been defined as a syndrome of reduced motor activity and spontaneity that can occur even when muscle stiffness and cogwheel rigidity are not observed and that can, at times, present clinically as a rather exact phenocopy of depression (Bermanzohn and Siris 1992; Martin et al. 1985; Rifkin et al. 1975, 1978; Siris 1987; Van Putten and May 1978). This phenocopy can include prominent blue mood, as well as anhedonia, pessimism, and reduced levels of subjective energy. The clinical differentiation of this state from depression may be almost impossible when it occurs in an insidious or subtle form, especially when large muscle extrapyramidal motor signs such as reduced arm swing or shuffling gait are not present (Siris 1987). Such patients may manifest simply a bump-on-a-log appearance, with little ability to initiate or sustain activity. This lack of energy and anhedonia may also be easily mistaken for negative symptoms of schizophrenia (see below), especially when motor stiffness affects the patients small muscles—in the face or vocal cords—which can cause the patient's appearance to be indistinguishable from that of blunted affect. Reduction of neuroleptic medication may partially protect patients from this form of akinesia, but it does not prevent its occurrence. Appropriate and aggressive treatment with antiparkinsonian medication may be required, often continuing into a sustained maintenance antiparkinsonian strategy (Manos et al. 1981a, 1981b). It is fortunate that neuroleptic-induced akinesia usually responds to adequate antiparkinsonian interventions rapidly—often within a few days to a week—so that relatively brief treatment trials can help make this differential diagnosis. However, it is essential to use adequate doses of antiparkinsonian agents to rule out akinesia. In general, with anticholinergic agents, this means gradually increasing the dose until either the symptoms resolve or side effects (e.g., blurry vision, dry mouth) appear. Usually, a full trial involves the equivalent of benztropine 6 mg/day in divided doses (Siris 1987).

Neuroleptic-induced akathisia. Akathisia can also present in a way that can easily be mistaken for a depressive syndrome. Although this motor restlessness syndrome is easily diagnosed as an extrapyramidal symptom in origin when it appears in its blatant form, more subtle variations that may be accompanied by dysphoric affect may present a very similar appearance to that of clinical depression (Siris 1985; Van Putten 1975). Although patients with akathisia may still be prone to behavioral excesses, the motor restlessness involved can easily be mistaken for the psychomotor agitation that frequently accompanies depression. Note that the dysphoria that can be associated with akathisia may be intense, and both suicidal ideation and suicidal behavior have been linked to this condition (Drake and Ehrlich 1985; Shear et al. 1983). In terms of treatment, minimizing the maintenance dose of a neuroleptic somewhat reduces the risk of akathisia, but this may be insufficient. Antiparkinsonian medications may be useful, but they are not as reliable for akathisia as they are for akinesia. Akathisia may also respond to the addition of a β-blocker or a benzodiazepine to the patient's neuroleptic regimen (Fleischhaker et al. 1990).

Negative Symptom Syndrome

The negative symptom syndrome of schizophrenia also has many features similar to those of depression (Andreasen and Olsen 1982; Bermanzohn and Siris 1992; Carpenter et al. 1985; Crow 1980; Kulhara et al. 1989; Siris et al. 1988a). The most prominent similarities between these conditions are anhedonia and lack of energy. Expression of affect, however, is most often useful in distinguishing these two conditions. Whereas depression is most frequently notable by the presence of a distinct sad mood, the negative symptom state is generally marked by blunted affect. Nevertheless, a clear cutoff between these clinical conditions is not necessarily apparent: negative symptom patients may be at least somewhat dysphoric, and depressed patients can have anhedonia that is more prominent than their degree of blue mood. From a pathophysiological perspective, the negative symptom state in schizophrenia has been hypothesized to involve a reduction in dopaminergic neurotransmission (Davis et al. 1991). Therefore, analogous to the above discussion regarding akinesia, neuroleptic medications could exacerbate this condition, and the minimum effective doses should therefore be employed. Otherwise, no clear-cut or well-established psychopharmacological intervention strategies exist specifically for negative symptoms. However, if the negative symptoms are secondary, rather than primarily due to a defect state, they may respond to antianxiety, antidepressant, or antiparkinsonian medications (Carpenter et al. 1985; Siris et al. 1988a).

Disappointment Reactions

Acute and chronic disappointment reactions are common in patients with schizophrenia and have several characteristics—especially dysphoria—in common with depression (Bartels and Drake 1988). Indeed, patients with schizophrenia often have much to be unhappy about in terms of their experiences. Operationally, a transient disappointment reaction can be distinguished from depression because the reaction is, by definition, transient and seldom lasts more than a week or two. In addition, a loss, stress, or disappointment is generally identifiable. No psychopharmacological intervention for transient disappointment reactions is indicated. Chronic disappointment reactions, often described as the *demoralization* syndrome (de Figueiredo 1993; Klein 1974), are often more difficult to distinguish from depression. Such syndromes generally occur in response to repeated discouragements or failures and are marked by apparent lack of initiative, a subjective sense of incompetence, and dysphoria. Again, no known psychopharmacological intervention is available, but it is important to recognize this condition because it might be amenable to more specific psychotherapeutic, psychosocial, or rehabilitative interventions.

Prodrome of Psychotic Relapse

Anecdotal studies that have monitored the course of patients with schizophrenia during intervals that included episodes of psychotic decompensation have often reported the emergence of symptoms reminiscent of depression before the outbreak of frank psychotic manifestations (Docherty et al. 1978; Green et al. 1990; Herz 1985; Herz and Melville 1980; Hirsch et al. 1989; Johnson 1988). Whether such depressive symptoms represent a reflection of underlying biological processes, a psychological reaction to the chain of events that is unfolding, or an epiphenomenological expression is unknown. Frequently, this stage of decompensation is also marked by other harbingers of impending relapse, such as social withdrawal, hypervigilance, anxiety, or idiosyncratic symptoms previously associated with psychotic relapse in the specific individual. Nevertheless, when depression-like features such as blue mood, guilt, low self-esteem, sleeplessness, anergia, impaired concentration, or indecisiveness are prominent, the definite identification of psychotic relapse can be difficult. Therefore, intensified nonspecific support and increased monitoring are the initial responses of choice when depressive symptoms emerge in the course of schizophrenia. Immediate reduction in neuroleptic medications may be premature and potentially counterproductive. Neuroleptics should only be reduced when it is clear that the schizophrenic patient's depression is stable and not a manifestation of an ongoing process of acute relapse.

Schizoaffective Disorder

The occurrence of depression in the course of schizophrenia raises the differential diagnostic question of schizoaffective disorder. Indeed, the boundary between associated depression in the course of schizophrenia and the existence of schizoaffective depression will depend on the exact set of operationalized criteria employed (Coryell et al. 1990; Levitt and Tsuang 1988; Taylor 1992), and it is critical to remember that none of these criteria are firmly based on a pathophysiological understanding of the conditions involved. According to the criteria that are currently most often used, a full affective syndrome must accompany a full manifestation of schizophrenic psychosis in order to diagnose schizoaffective disorder. A comprehensive exposition of the treatment of schizoaffective disorder is a topic unto itself (Levitt and Tsuang 1988; Siris 1993; Siris and Lavin 1995). Within this domain, however, fewer studies have been undertaken of schizoaffective depression than of schizoaffective mania. In the former category, an insufficient number of studies have been performed to create clear-cut guidelines for treatment. Neuroleptics appear to be the agents of choice for acute treatment of schizoaffective depressions when the patient is floridly psychotic. At other phases of the illness, there may be a role for lithium, electroconvulsive therapy, or adjunctive antidepressant agents added to the neuroleptic; the latter strategy probably would be restricted to a more chronic phase of the disorder when the psychosis is relatively quiescent in comparison to the depressive manifestations.

Adjunctive Treatment Strategies

Antidepressant Medications

When associated syndromes of depression occur in patients with schizophrenia who are not flagrantly psychotic, and when the differential diagnoses of impending psychotic relapse, transient disappointment reaction, and neuroleptic-induced akinesia and akathisia have been ruled out, a question sensibly arises about the potential benefit of adding an antidepressant medication to the patient's best adjusted neuroleptic dose. Several careful studies have examined this question, and these studies have been reviewed (Plasky 1991; Siris 1991). In summary, the results of these studies are cautiously positive. Studies that used doses of antidepressant agents comparable to those used in the treatment of primary depression and that included treatment trials of 6 weeks or longer had better results than those trials that did not. In addition, trials among outpatients had superior outcomes compared with trials among inpatients. In regard to this last observation, it is unclear whether the relevant issue concerned outpatients' underlying conditions or whether the supports and expectations of the outpatient setting constituted a superior venue for a favorable response to an antidepressant agent. The most successful antidepressant trial increased the dose of adjunctive antidepressant gradually to its full therapeutic level (i.e., adjunctive imipramine in weekly increments of 50 mg/day to a final dose of 200 mg/day) (Siris et al. 1987). This gradual increase is consistent with the notion that patients with schizophrenia react as if they are "brittle," and sudden changes may therefore be difficult for them, whether they are psychopharmacological, psychological, or social. Furthermore, in the context of a gradual increase in the antidepressant dose, it was possible to maintain these patients on their full dosage of antiparkinsonian medications without undue exacerbation of anticholinergic side effects, and the inclusion of the antiparkinsonian medication may have also contributed to the positive outcomes in those patients who responded (Siris et al. 1983).

Specific "head-to-head" comparisons of the efficacy of different antidepressant agents as adjuncts in the treatment of depression in patients with schizophrenia have not been reported. It is therefore difficult to conclude whether there is a preferred agent. Those positive studies that have been reported have tended to employ older and biochemically "dirtier" tricyclic antidepressant agents. Randomized, double-blind studies of adjunctive use of specific serotonin reuptake inhibitor drugs for this patient population have not as yet been reported, although this may be because those drugs were more recently released. Additionally, monoamine oxidase inhibitor antidepressants have not been adequately investigated in depressed patients with schizophrenia, so there is no basis for making recommendations concerning these agents. On the other hand, it may be pertinent to note that evidence suggests that at least some monoamine oxidase inhibitors may be useful adjunctive agents in schizophrenic patients with negative symptom syndromes (Bodkin et al. 1992; Bucci 1987; Perenyi et al. 1992)—possibly not an unrelated situation, as noted in the above section, "Negative Symptom Syndrome."

Data on continuation and maintenance treatment with adjunctive antidepressant agents have been limited. One randomized, double-blind study, however, indicated that such maintenance treatment helped avert long-term depressive relapse in patients who had initially responded favorably in an acute treatment trial for postpsychotic depression (Siris et al. 1994). It is interesting that the patients in that study who were maintained on adjunctive antidepressants also had fewer psychotic exacerbations, although it is unclear to what extent firm conclusions can be drawn from this highly selective population.

Lithium

The majority of studies concerning the use of adjunctive lithium in patients with schizophrenia have focused on the control of acute episodes of psychosis rather than on lithium's possible effect on symptoms of depression (Christison et al. 1991; Plasky 1991). Indeed, excitement, overactivity, and euphoria are usually mentioned as positive prognosticators of lithium responsiveness, along with a history of previous affective episodes, an overall episodic course, and a history of family members with affective disorders. However, depression has been specifically mentioned at least once as a favorable prognosticator for adjunctive lithium in schizophrenia (Lerner et al. 1988). It is therefore rational to attempt a trial of adjunctive lithium in schizophrenic patients with depression who are unresponsive to, or intolerant of, adjunctive antidepressant medication. Although specific studies are lacking to substantiate this theory, the doses and blood levels of lithium to be tested would logically be the same as those utilized in patients with affective disorders. Lithium could also be evaluated as an augmentation strategy for patients with schizophrenia who do not respond to adjunctive antidepressants—again on an empirical basis without a published study to support this use.

Benzodiazepines

As an adjunctive treatment in schizophrenia, benzodiazepines have usually been studied or advocated in the treatment of acute psychosis, excessive anxiety, or negative symptoms (Christison et al. 1991; Kellner et al. 1975; Wolkowitz and Pickar 1991), although even for these conditions conclusions about their ultimate utility are somewhat divided. Nevertheless, because course-related dysphoria in schizophrenia may represent a combination of anxiety and depression (Norman and Malla 1991), some schizophrenic patients with depressive symptoms may improve on a trial of an adjunctive benzodiazepine (Pato et al. 1989; Wolkowitz and Pickar 1991). Also, as noted above, the addition of a benzodiazepine to the regimen of patients with dysphoria attributable to akathisia may be beneficial (Fleischhaker et al. 1990; Sachdev and Lonergan 1991). Any such trial of adjunctive benzodiazepines is, of course, empirical, and continuing treatment should be based on ongoing results. The potentially sedative and habit-forming nature of benzodiazepines should be considered. Nevertheless, the continuing use of benzodiazepines is justified in those patients who clearly show relief of symptoms or enhanced functioning.

Psychosocial Interventions

The potential value of psychosocial interventions among depressed schizophrenic patients deserves emphasis. Although the benefit of such treatments in these patients has generally not been documented with controlled studies (which would be enormously difficult to do and prohibitively expensive), clinical experience and patient self-reports support the usefulness of organized supportive interventions such as skill building, stress reduction, problem solving, and psychoeducation. Appropriate rehabilitative techniques (Anthony and Liberman 1986) include components that enhance self-confidence and improve self-esteem so that patients acquire abilities valuable for everyday living, learning, working, and socializing. To evaluate these interventions, future research must determine whether improved functioning leads to better mood or whether improved mood leads to enhanced functioning, or whether these dimensions are independent of each other.

Conclusion

The appearance of a depression-like syndrome is common in the longitudinal course of schizophrenia, and it can be associated with substantial morbidity. The approach to treatment entails a careful differential diagnosis, the results of which will suggest appropriate psychopharmacological and other interventions. Ultimately, because each patient is different and the recommendations of science are still less than exact, the patient's final treatment plan must be empirically derived, based on the outcomes of a logical sequence of interventions.

References

Andreasen NC, Olsen S: Negative symptoms in schizophrenia: definition and reliability. Arch Gen Psychiatry 39:789–794, 1982

Anthony WA, Liberman RP: The practice of psychiatric rehabilitation: historical, conceptual and research base. Schizophr Bull 12:542–559, 1986

Bandelow B, Muller P, Gaebel W, et al: Depressive syndromes in schizophrenic patients after discharge from hospital. Eur Arch Psychiatry Clin Neurosci 240:113–120, 1991

Barnes TR, Curson DA, Liddle PF, et al: The nature and prevalence of depression in chronic schizophrenic in-patients. Br J Psychiatry 154:486–491, 1989

Bartels SJ, Drake RE: Depressive symptoms in schizophrenia: comprehensive differential diagnosis. Compr Psychiatry 29:467–483, 1988

Bartels SJ, Drake RE: Depression in schizophrenia: current guidelines to treatment. Psychiatr Q 60:337–357, 1989

Bermanzohn PC, Siris SG: Akinesia: a syndrome common to parkinsonism, retarded depression, and negative symptoms. Compr Psychiatry 33:221–232, 1992

Berrios GE, Bulbena A: Post psychotic depression: the Fulbourn cohort. Acta Psychiatr Scand 76:89–93, 1987

Bodkin A, Cannon S, Cohen B, et al: Selegiline treatment of negative symptoms of schizophrenia and schizoaffective disorder. Abstracts of panels and posters presented at the 31st annual meeting of the American College of Neuropsychopharmacology, San Juan, Puerto Rico, December 14–18, 1992

Breier A, Schreiber JL, Dyer J, et al: National Institute of Mental Health longitudinal study of chronic schizophrenia: prognosis and predictors of outcome. Arch Gen Psychiatry 48:239–246, 1991

Bucci L: The negative symptoms of schizophrenia and the monoamine oxidase inhibitors. Psychopharmacology (Berl) 91:104–108, 1987

Caldwell CB, Gottesman II: Schizophrenics kill themselves too: a review of risk factors for suicide. Schizophr Bull 16:571–589, 1990

Carpenter WT Jr, Heinrichs DW, Alphs LD: Treatment of negative symptoms. Schizophr Bull 11:440–452, 1985

Carpenter WT Jr, Heinrichs DW, Hanlon TE: A comparative trial of pharmacologic strategies in schizophrenia. Am J Psychiatry 144:1466–1470, 1987

Christison GW, Kirch DG, Wyatt RJ: When symptoms persist: choosing among alternative somatic treatments for schizophrenia. Schizophr Bull 17:217–245, 1991

Coryell W, Keller M, Lavori P, et al: Affective syndromes, psychotic features, and prognosis, I: depression. Arch Gen Psychiatry 47:651–657, 1990

Crow TJ: Molecular pathology of schizophrenia: more than one disease process? BMJ 280:66–68, 1980

Davis KL, Kahn RS, Ko G, et al: Dopamine in schizophrenia: a review and reconceptualization. Am J Psychiatry 148:1474–1486, 1991

DeAlarcon R, Carney MWP: Severe depressive mood changes following slow-release intramuscular fluphenazine injection. BMJ 3:564–567, 1969

de Figueiredo JM: Depression and demoralization: phenomenologic differences and research perspectives. Compr Psychiatry 34:308–311, 1993

Docherty JP, van Kammen DP, Siris SG, et al: Stages of onset of schizophrenic psychosis. Am J Psychiatry 135:420–426, 1978

Drake RE, Ehrlich J: Suicide attempts associated with akathisia. Am J Psychiatry 142:499–501, 1985

Fleischhaker WW, Roth SD, Kane JM: The pharmacologic treatment of neuroleptic-induced akathisia. J Clin Psychopharmacol 10:12–21, 1990

Floru L, Heinrich K, Wittek F: The problem of post-psychotic schizophrenic depressions and their pharmacological induction. International Pharmacopsychiatry 10:230–239, 1975

Galdi J, Reider RO, Silber D, et al: Genetic factors in the response to neuroleptics in schizophrenia: a pharmacogenetic study. Psychol Med 11:713–728, 1981

Green MF, Nuechterlein KH, Ventura J, et al: The temporal relationship between depressive and psychotic symptoms in recent-onset schizophrenia. Am J Psychiatry 147:179–182, 1990

Harrow M, Potter CA, Sands JF, et al: Depression in schizophrenia at a 4.5 year follow-up: are neuroleptics, akinesia, or anhedonia involved? Paper presented at the 146th annual meeting of the American Psychiatric Association, San Francisco, CA, May 1993

Herz M: Prodromal symptoms and prevention of relapse in schizophrenia. J Clin Psychiatry 46 (11 sect 2):22–25, 1985

Herz M, Melville C: Relapse in schizophrenia. Am J Psychiatry 137:801–805, 1980

Herz MI, Glazer WM, Mostert MA, et al: Intermittent vs maintenance medication in schizophrenia: two year results. Arch Gen Psychiatry 48:333–339, 1991

Hirsch SR, Gaind R, Rohde PD, et al: Outpatient maintenance of chronic schizophrenic patients with long-acting fluphenazine: double-blind placebo trial. BMJ 1:633–637, 1973

Hirsch SR, Jolley AG, Barnes TRE, et al: Dysphoric and depressive symptoms in chronic schizophrenia. Schizophr Res 2:259–264, 1989

Hogarty GE, Munetz MR: Pharmacogenic depression among outpatient schizophrenic patients: a failure to substantiate. J Clin Psychopharmacol 4:17–24, 1984

Hogarty GE, McEvoy JP, Munetz M, et al: Dose of fluphenazine, familial expressed emotion, and outcome in schizophrenia: results of a two-year controlled study. Arch Gen Psychiatry 45:797–805, 1988

Johnson DAW: Depressions in schizophrenia: some observations on prevalence, etiology, and treatment. Acta Psychiatr Scand 63 (suppl 291):137–144, 1981

Johnson DAW: The significance of depression in the prediction of relapse in chronic schizophrenia. Br J Psychiatry 152:320–323, 1988

Jolley AG, Hirsch SR: Brief intermittent neuroleptic prophylaxis for stable schizophrenic outpatients: two year outcome. Schizophr Res 2:208, 1989

Kane JM, Rifkin A, Woerner M, et al: Low-dose neuroleptic treatment of outpatient schizophrenics, I: preliminary results for relapse rates. Arch Gen Psychiatry 40:893–896, 1983

Kellner R, Wilson RM, Mildawer MD, et al: Anxiety in schizophrenia: the responses to chlordiazepoxide in an intensive design study. Arch Gen Psychiatry 32:1246–1254, 1975

Klein DF: Endogenomorphic depression: a conceptual and terminological revision. Arch Gen Psychiatry 31:447–454, 1974

Knights A, Hirsch SR: 'Revealed' depression and drug treatment for schizophrenia. Arch Gen Psychiatry 38:806–811, 1981

Kulhara P, Avasthi A, Chadda R, et al: Negative and depressive symptoms in schizophrenia. Br J Psychiatry 154:207–211, 1989

Leff J, Tress K, Edwards B: The clinical course of depressive symptoms in schizophrenia. Schizophr Res 1:25–30, 1988

Lerner Y, Mintzer Y, Schestatzky M: Lithium combined with haloperidol in schizophrenic patients. Br J Psychiatry 153:359–362, 1988

Levitt JJ, Tsuang MT: The heterogeneity of schizoaffective disorder: implications for treatment. Am J Psychiatry 145:926–936, 1988

Manos N, Gkiouzepas J, Logothetis J: The need for continuous use of antiparkinsonian medication with chronic schizophrenic patients receiving long-term neuroleptic therapy. Am J Psychiatry 138:184–188, 1981a

Manos N, Gkiouzepas J, Tzotzoras T, et al: Gradual withdrawal of antiparkinson medication in chronic schizophrenics: any better than the abrupt? J Nerv Ment Dis 169:659–661, 1981b
Marder SR, Van Putten T, Mintz J, et al: Low- and conventional-dose maintenance therapy with fluphenazine decanoate: two-year outcome. Arch Gen Psychiatry 44:518–521, 1987
Martin RL, Cloninger RC, Guze SB, et al: Frequency and differential diagnosis of depressive syndromes in schizophrenia. J Clin Psychiatry 46 (11 sect 2):9–13, 1985
McGlashan TH, Carpenter WT Jr: Postpsychotic depression in schizophrenia. Arch Gen Psychiatry 33:231–239, 1976
Moller HJ, von Zerssen D: Depressive states occurring during the neuroleptic treatment of schizophrenia. Schizophr Bull 8:109–117, 1982
Moller HJ, von Zerssen D: Depression in schizophrenia, in Handbook of Studies on Schizophrenia. Edited by Burrows GD, Norman TR, Rubinstein G. Amsterdam, Elsevier, 1986, pp 183–191
Norman RM, Malla AK: Dysphoric mood and symptomatology in schizophrenia. Psychol Med 21:897–903, 1991
Pato CN, Wolkowitz OM, Rapaport M, et al: Benzodiazepine augmentation of neuroleptic treatment in patients with schizophrenia. Psychopharmacol Bull 25:263–266, 1989
Perenyi A, Goswami U, Frecska E, et al: L-deprenyl in treating negative symptoms of schizophrenia (letter). Psychiatry Res 42:189–191, 1992
Plasky P: Antidepressant usage in schizophrenia. Schizophr Bull 17:649–657, 1991
Rifkin A, Quitkin F, Klein DF: Akinesia: a poorly recognized drug-induced extrapyramidal behavioral disorder. Arch Gen Psychiatry 32:672–674, 1975
Rifkin A, Quitkin F, Kane J, et al: Are prophylactic antiparkinsonian drugs necessary? A controlled study of procyclidine withdrawal. Arch Gen Psychiatry 35:483–489, 1978
Roy A: Do neuroleptics cause depression? Biol Psychiatry 19:777–781, 1984
Roy A: Depression, attempted suicide, and suicide in patients with chronic schizophrenia. Psychiatr Clin North Am 9:193–206, 1986
Roy A, Thompson R, Kennedy S: Depression in chronic schizophrenia. Br J Psychiatry 142:465–470, 1983
Sachdev P, Lonergan C: The present status of akathisia. J Nerv Ment Dis 179:381–391, 1991
Shear K, Francis A, Wieden P: Suicide associated with akathisia and depot fluphenazine treatment. J Clin Psychopharmacol 3:235–236, 1983
Shuwall MA, Siris SG: Suicidal ideation in post-psychotic depression. Compr Psychiatry 35:132–134, 1994

Siris SG: Akathisia and "acting-out." J Clin Psychiatry 46:395–397, 1985

Siris SG: Akinesia and post-psychotic depression: a difficult differential diagnosis. J Clin Psychiatry 48:240–243, 1987

Siris SG: Diagnosis of secondary depression in schizophrenia: implications for DSM-IV. Schizophr Bull 17:75–98, 1991

Siris SG: The treatment of schizoaffective disorder, in Current Psychiatric Therapy. Edited by Dunner DL. Philadelphia, PA, WB Saunders, 1993, pp 160–165

Siris SG, Lavin M: Schizoaffective disorder, schizophreniform disorder, and acute psychotic disorder, in Comprehensive Textbook of Psychiatry, 6th Edition. Edited by Kaplan HI, Sadock BJ. Baltimore, MD, Williams & Wilkins, 1995, pp 1019–1031

Siris SG, Harmon GK, Endicott J: Post-psychotic depressive symptoms in hospitalized schizophrenic patients. Arch Gen Psychiatry 38:1122–1123, 1981

Siris SG, Rifkin A, Reardon GT, et al: Comparative side effects to imipramine, benztropine, or their combination, in patients receiving fluphenazine decanoate. Am J Psychiatry 140:1069–1071, 1983

Siris SG, Morgan V, Fagerstrom R, et al: Adjunctive imipramine in the treatment of post-psychotic depression: a controlled trial. Arch Gen Psychiatry 44:533–539, 1987

Siris SG, Adan F, Cohen M, et al: Post-psychotic depression and negative symptoms: an investigation of syndromal overlap. Am J Psychiatry 145:1532–1537, 1988a

Siris SG, Strahan A, Mandeli J, et al: Fluphenazine decanoate dose and severity of depression in patients with post-psychotic depressions. Schizophr Res 1:31–35, 1988b

Siris SG, Bermanzohn PC, Mason SE, et al: Maintenance imipramine therapy for secondary depression in schizophrenia: a controlled trial. Arch Gen Psychiatry 51:109–115, 1994

Strian F, Heger R, Klicpera C: The time structure of depressive mood in schizophrenic patients. Acta Psychiatr Scand 65:66–73, 1982

Szymanski HV, Simon JC, Gutterman N: Recovery from schizophrenic psychosis. Am J Psychiatry 140:335–338, 1983

Taylor MA: Are schizophrenia and affective disorder related? A selective literature review. Am J Psychiatry 149:22–32, 1992

Van Putten T: The many faces of akathisia. Compr Psychiatry 16:43–47, 1975

Van Putten T, May PRA: 'Akinetic depression' in schizophrenia. Arch Gen Psychiatry 35:1101–1107, 1978

Wise RA: Neuroleptics and operant behavior: the anhedonia hypothesis. Behavioral and Brain Sciences 5:39–87, 1982

Wistedt B, Palmstierna T: Depressive symptoms in chronic schizophrenic patients after withdrawal of long-acting neuroleptics. J Clin Psychiatry 44:369–371, 1983

Wolkowitz OM, Pickar D: Benzodiazepines in the treatment of schizophrenia: a review and reappraisal. Am J Psychiatry 148:714–726, 1991

Conclusion

Alan Breier, M.D.

One of the most important implications, for patients and their families, resulting from the developments reviewed in this volume is optimism for the future. The therapeutic goals of the past "neuroleptic era" were rather modest and included maintaining stability in the community and suppressing the most florid symptomatology, even though overall quality of life may have been poor and the chronic negative and positive symptoms that persisted in many patients caused social isolation and psychic pain. The advent of a new era in the pharmacotherapy of schizophrenia marked by new antipsychotic agents, strategies with better side-effect profiles, and the promise of many novel agents in the near future encourages more ambitious therapeutic goals. Future treatment goals for patients with schizophrenia will focus on restoring a high quality of life; achieving gainful employment and meaningful social relationships; substantially reducing symptoms; and, more than ever before, eliminating chronic negative and positive symptoms and other debilitating features of this illness. In short, the treatment philosophy will shift toward the goal of recovery.

One example of the short-term impact of widespread use of the new atypical antipsychotic drugs is a significant reduction in, and conceivably the ultimate elimination of, extrapyramidal side effects. This alone would likely result in improved compliance (because akathisia and other neuroleptic-induced side effects are often responsible for patients' decisions to stop taking neuroleptics), with consequent fewer relapses and related hospitalizations. Moreover, extrapyramidal side effects mimic negative symptoms and may impair quality of life; thus, these psychopathological domains may improve.

I believe that there is now more reason for hope and optimism for the treatment of schizophrenia than at any other time in the therapeutic history of this illness. Critical to the continued success of this "new pharmacotherapy of schizophrenia" are advances in research and education. Increased emphasis on psychotropic drug development and progress in the understanding of the pathophysiology of this illness are needed. Once new therapeutic agents are available, it will be important to educate clinicians about their use and encourage a rapid transition to the newer compounds. It will be necessary to prioritize this effort at the national level with a strong commitment of funds and resources.

Index

Page numbers printed in **boldface** *type refer to tables or figures.*

Abnormal Involuntary Movements Scale (AIMS), 143, **145**
Adjunctive treatment
  for depression
    antidepressants, 212–214
    benzodiazepines, 214–215
    lithium, 214
    social interventions, 215
  goals of, 154
Affective symptoms, risperidone for, 30–31
Age, clozapine-induced agranulocytosis and, 10–11
Aggression, *vs.* refractory psychosis, 108
Agranulocytosis, clozapine-induced, 2, 3, 10–11
AIMS (Abnormal Involuntary Movements Scale), 143, **145**
AJ76, 72, **73**, **77**
AJ-119, **73**
Akathisia
  neuroleptic dosages and, 93, 94, 95, 96–97
  propranolol for, 114, 139
  vs. depression, 209
Akinesia
  neuroleptic dosage and, 94, 95, 96–97
  vs. depression, 208–209
α_2 antagonism, 62, 146
Alprazolam
  adjunctive, 159
  augmentation, 165
    case reports of, 168–170
    for treatment-resistant patients, 155–156
  potency of, **160**
  withdrawal, 168–169
Alternative therapy. *See* Adjunctive treatment
Amisulpride, **77**
Amitriptyline, 190–191
Amperozide
  antipsychotic efficacy, 18, 47–48
  mechanism of action, 48, **77**
  plus neuroleptics, 119
  side effects, 48

Amphetamine
clinical trial, 185–186
dopaminergic activity, 118, 123, 185
for negative symptoms, 123
Anticholinergics, for negative symptoms, 191–192
Anticonvulsants
indications for, 113
phenytoin, for clozapine-induced seizures, 11
for positive symptoms, 110–113
Antidepressants. *See also* Tricyclic antidepressants (TCAs)
adjunctive, 182–183, 212–214
for depression, 123, 212–214
for negative symptoms, 120–121, 182–183
plus neuroleptics, 59, 61
Antidipsotropic agents, 121
Antidopaminergic drugs
anatomically selective D_2 antagonists, 69–70
cotransmitter modulation and, 67–68
drug development strategies, 63, **64**
partial dopamine agonists, 63–67, **65**
selective D_4- or D_3-receptor blockade, 70–72, **70**
Antiparkinsonian agents
extrapyramidal side effects and, 34, 94
for neuroleptic-induced akathisia, 209
for neuroleptic-induced akinesia, 208–209
Antipsychotics
atypical, 16
benefits of, 223–224
preclinical screen for, 43
benefit-to-risk issues, 102
disadvantages of, 15
dosage, 92–95
drug development. *See* Drug development
efficacy of, 43, 91
future new, goals for, 42–44, **42**
for maintenance treatment, 96–99
new, 44–45, **44**
amperozide, 47–48
olanzapine, 46
remoxipride, 48–49
risperidone, **44**, 45
seroquel, 47
sertindole, 45–46
for refractory patients, 95–96
selection of, 91–92
side effects of, 91
Apomorphine, 64–65, **73**
Augmentation agents
algorithm for, 106–107, **107**
benzodiazepines, 116, 158–159
β-blockers, 113–115

calcium channel blockers, 116
carbamazepine, 110–112
idazoxan, 141–146, **142, 144, 145**
lithium, 108–110
noradrenergic agents, 117
reserpine, 115
treatment decisions, 122–123
valproic acid, 110, 112–113

Benserazide, plus L-dopa, 184–185
Benzodiazepines
abuse or dependence, 166
adjunctive, 158–159
dose and, 162, **162**
response specificity and, 163–164, **163,** 167
for akathisia, 209
anxiolytic effects, 155
case reports, 167–170
clinical guidelines/ considerations, 165–167, **168**
clinical response, 160, 167
comparison of, 160–161, **160**
dose and, 162, **162,** 167
onset/duration of, 161–162, 167
pharmacokinetic interactions and, 163
plasma level and, 163
predictors of, 165, 166
specificity of, 163–164, **163**
variability of, 165, 166
dopamine neurotransmission and, 155–156
dose-response relationship, 162, **162**
GABA neurotransmission and, 156
indications for, 116
literature review, 157–158
for negative symptoms, 183
rationale for usage, 155–157
side effects, 165
as sole agent, 158
Benztropine plus fluphenazine, augmentation with idazoxan, 141–143, **142**
β-Blockers
for akathisia, 209
for positive symptoms, 113–115
side effects, 114–115
B-HT 920, 67, **77**
Bipolar disorder, 5–6, 106
BMY 14802, 76
Borderline personality disorder, 106
Brief Psychiatric Rating Scale (BPRS)
anergia factor score
amitriptyline and, 190–191
bromocriptine and, 186
clozapine and, 193, 194
mianserin and, 191
risperidone and, 195
ritanserin and, 190

Brief Psychiatric Rating Scale (BPRS) *(continued)*
clozapine *vs.* chlorpromazine, 3–4
L-dopa adjunctive treatment and, 184
fluphenazine decanoate and, 97
ICI 204,636 (Seroquel) and, 47
idazoxan plus fluphenazine, 143, **144, 145**
risperidone and, 31
risperidone long-term studies, 36
total score, ritanserin and, 190
Bromocriptine, 65, 118, 123, 186
Bunney-Hamburg Global Rating Scales, 142–143, **145**

Caffeine, 207
Calcium channel blockers, 116, 123
Camazepam, **160**
Canadian clinical trial, 32–35
Carbamazepine, 110–112
Carbidopa plus L-dopa, 185
β-Carbolines, 156
Catalepsy, 18, 43, 49
CF 25397, 65
Chlordiazepoxide, **160**
Chlorpromazine
binding profile, **60**, 72
discovery of, 1, 2
dopamine receptor selectivity, **73**
dosage, 92–93
negative symptoms and, 164
vs. clozapine, 3–4, 8, 11, 193
vs. lithium, 108–109
vs. remoxipride, 196
Cholecystokinin (CCK-8), 67
Cholinergic hypothesis of negative symptoms, 191
CKK-8 (cholecystokinin), 67
Clinical psychopharmacological research, 89–90. *See also* Drug development
Clomipramine, for negative symptoms, 120–121
Clonazepam, **160**
Clonidine, **134**, 138
Clozapine
agranulocytosis, 2, 3
incidence of, 10–11
predictors of, 10–11
α_2 antagonism, 62
binding profile, **60**
broad receptor blockade and, 59
dopamine receptor binding, 6, 58–59, 193
D_2 affinity, 62–63, **73**
D_4 affinity and, 63, 72, **73**
efficacy, 43, **44**, 57, 137
vs. chlorpromazine, 3–4, 193
vs. haloperidol, 3, 4–5, 8–10, 193
FDA approval of, 4, **44**
history of, 2–3
indications, 4–6

length of trial, adequate, 8, **9**
mechanism of action, 16, **77**
multicenter trial, 3–4
for negative symptoms, 8–10, 192–194, 197
noradrenergic effects, 141
norepinephrine and, 140, 146–147
normetanephrine and, 140
plasma levels, 8
plus disulfiram, 121
predictors of clinical improvement and, 7–8
responder rates, in chronic schizophrenia, 6–7, **7**
selectivity of, **73**
serotonin-receptor antagonism and, 119, 189
side effects, 2, 3, 10–11
Cocaine abuse, 121–122
Compliance, 153
Conceptual disorganization. *See* Positive symptoms
Cotransmitter modulation, 67–68
CP 99994, 68
D-Cycloserine, 120
Cyproheptadine, 16, 17, 119

D_1 antagonism, 61–62
D_2 antagonists
anatomically selective, 69–70
in combination therapy, 59, 61–62
limitations of, 15
serum prolactin and, 35
D_4 blockers, 51

Deinstitutionalism, 1
Delusions. *See* Positive symptoms
Demoralization syndrome, 210–211
L-Deprenyl, 187
Depression
adjunctive treatment strategies, 212–215
diagnosis, importance of, 205
differential diagnosis
disappointment reactions and, 210–211
extrapyramidal side effects and, 208–209
negative symptom syndrome and, 210
neuroleptic-induced dysphoria and, 207–208
organic factors and, 206–207
prodrome of psychotic relapse and, 211
schizoaffective disorder and, 211–212
drug-induced, 206
incidence, 205
secondary, 137
treatment, 215–216
Depressogenic drugs, 206
Desipramine, 121–122, 123
Diazepam, **160**
Diltiazem, 116

Disappointment reactions,
vs. depression, 210–211
Disulfiram, 121
L-Dopa
dopaminergic activity, 118, 123
for negative symptoms, 123, 184–185
Dopamine
lithium effects on, 109
neurotransmission, benzodiazepines and, 155–156
prefrontal cortical system, 156–157
Dopamine agonists
intrinsic activity, **65**
for negative symptoms, 184–187
partial, 63–67, **65**
Dopamine hypothesis, 117, 134, 184
Dopamine receptor blockade. *See also* D_2 antagonists
D_1, 61–62
D_3-selective, 70–72
D_4-selective, 70–72
selective combinations of, 59, 61–62
with serotonin-receptor antagonism, 61–62
Dopamine receptors
clozapine and, 16
D_2, 6
as autoreceptor, 64
localization of, 71
low affinity, drugs with, 62–63
risperidone affinity for, 20
D_3, 64, 71–72
D_4, 51
clozapine affinity for, 63
localization of, 71
Dopaminergic agents. *See also specific dopaminergic agents*
D_4- and D_2-receptor selectivity, **73**
for negative symptoms, 117–118, 123
psychosis induced by, 6
Dosage. *See also under specific drugs*
for conventional neuroleptic treatment, 92–95
requirements, for maintenance treatment, 97
strategies, 102
Drug development
serendipity and, 58
strategies, 58
hypothetical experimental, 72–76
novel antidopaminergic, 63–72
refined clozapine-like, 58–63
strategies for, 50–53
Dysphoria
neuroleptic-induced, *vs.* depression, 207–208
secondary negative symptoms, 182–183

EMD 49980, **77**
Epinephrine, **134**

EPS. *See* Extrapyramidal side effects (EPS)
ESRS (Extrapyramidal Symptom Rating Scale), 34
Estazolam, **160**
Excitement. *See* Positive symptoms
Extrapyramidal side effects (EPS). *See also* Akathisia; Akinesia; Tardive dyskinesia
  amperozide and, 48
  atypical antipsychotics and, 16
  clozapine and, 9, 193, 194
  dosage and, 93–94
  dosage-reduction strategies and, 101
  future new antipsychotics and, 42–43
  incidence, 102
  lack of, as goal for future new antipsychotics, 42–43
  maintenance dosage and, 97
  neuroleptics and, 1, 2
  noncompliance and, 97
  prophylactic antiparkinsonian agents and, 94
  risperidone and, 33–35
  vs. depression, 208–209
Extrapyramidal Symptom Rating Scale (ESRS), 34

Fenfluramine, for negative symptoms, 189–190
Fifteen-nation trial, 30, 32–33, **33**, 34–35
Fluoxetine, for negative symptoms, 120–121, 190
Flupentixol decanoate, 98
Fluphenazine
  augmentation, with alprazolam, 168–169
  dosages, 94–95
  plasma levels, **145**
  plus benztropine, augmentation with idazoxan, 141–143, **142**
  plus idazoxan, 51
  refractory patients and, 96
Fluphenazine decanoate
  augmentation, with alprazolam, 169–170
  maintenance treatment, 97–98
  targeted or intermittent treatment, 100
Fluvoxamine, for negative symptoms, 120–121, 190

GABA (γ-Aminobutyric acid), 156
GABA hypothesis, 156
γ-Aminobutyric acid (GABA), 156
Glutamate, 51
Glutamatergic agents, 51–52, 74–75
Glycine, 75
G protein, 146
G protein–coupled receptor, 70–71, **70**
G-protein coupling, 71
G-protein effectors, 52
Grandiosity. *See* Positive symptoms

Hallucinations. *See* Positive symptoms
Haloperidol
  binding profile, **60**
  blood levels, carbamazepine and, 111–112
  clinical global improvement and, 26, **27**
  dopamine receptor selectivity, **73**
  dosages, 94–95
  extrapyramidal side effects and, 33–34
  North American multicenter study, 26, 27, **27–29**
  plus alprazolam, 159, 163
  plus cyproheptadine, 17
  plus lithium, 109
  plus ritanserin, 17, 61
  receptor-binding profile, **19**
  refractory patients and, 96
  social behavior and, 164
  vs. clozapine, 3, 4–5, 8–11, 193
  vs. remoxipride, 48–49, 196
  vs. risperidone
    Canadian clinical trials, 32, 33, 34
    Fifteen-nation trial, 30, 32–33, **33**
    North American double-blind trial, 26–34, **27–33**
High-potency neuroleptics. *See also* Fluphenazine; Haloperidol
  efficacy, 92
  high dosages of, 93
  side effects of, 182
Homovanillic acid, 156, 157
Hospitalization
  clozapine and, 5
  targeted treatment and, 100
Hostility. *See* Positive symptoms
5-HT_2 blocking agents. *See* Serotonin receptor antagonists
9-Hydroxyrisperidone (9-OH), 20–21
Hyperdopaminergic agents, 50
Hypotheses of schizophrenia, 72–73

ICI 204,636 (Seroquel), 47
Idazoxan
  augmentation therapy, 141–146, **142, 144, 145**
    with fluphenazine, 51
    with haloperidol, 62
  chemical structure, **134**
  efficacy, 117
Imipramine, for negative symptoms, 188–189
Injectable or decanoate preparations, 106
Intermittent therapy, 99–101, 139–140

Ketamine, 74

Lithium
  adjunctive, 59, 214
  contraindications, 110
  dosages, 110
  for psychosis, 108–109
  side effects, 109–110
Lorazepam, **160,** 162
Low-potency neuroleptics, 182. *See also* Chlorpromazine
Loxapine, dopamine receptor selectivity, **73**
Lysergic acid diethylamide (LSD), 20

Maintenance treatment, 96–99
MAOIs. *See* Monoamine oxidase inhibitors (MAOIs)
Maprotiline, for negative symptoms, 188–189
Mazindol
  for comorbid substance abuse, 121–122, 123
  dopamine reuptake and, 186
  side effects, 118
Melperone, dopamine receptor selectivity, **73**
Metabotropic receptors, 70–71, **70**
Methadone, 122
3-Methoxy-4-hydroxyphenylglycol (MHPG), 135
Methylphenidate, 118
MHPG (3-methoxy-4-hydroxyphenylglycol), 135
Mianserin
  antipsychotic efficacy, 18
  BPRS anergia factor score and, 191
  for negative symptoms, 190–191
  serotonin receptor blockade, 16
Milacemide
  antipsychotic efficacy, lack of, 52, 75, 119–120
  for negative symptoms, 52
Monoamine oxidase, 186
Monoamine oxidase inhibitors (MAOIs)
  adjunctive, 213
  for negative symptoms, 120, 186–187
Motor disturbances, benzodiazepines and, 164
Multiple personality disorder, 106

Naltrexone, 121
National Institute of Mental Health Longitudinal Study of Chronic Schizophrenia, 153
NE100, 76
Negative symptoms
  in acute treatment phase, 90, 91
  cholinergic hypothesis of, 191
  conceptual models, 180
  with depression, 137
  differential diagnosis, 180
  historical aspects, 180
  neuroleptics and, 153, 223

Negative symptoms *(continued)*
North American multicenter trial, 195
secondary
to antipsychotic medication, 181–182
to dysphoric affect, 182–183
to psychotic symptoms, 181
vs. primary, 180
social/occupational impairments and, 179
syndrome, *vs.* depression, 210
treatment
anticholinergics for, 191–192
antidepressants for, 120–121
atypical antipsychotics for, 192–197
benzodiazepines for, 164, 183
clozapine for, 8–10, 192–194
dopamine agonists for, 184–187
dopaminergic agents, 117–118
evaluation of, 183–184
first-line augmentation agents for, 123
future new antipsychotics and, 43
glycine for, 119–120
idazoxan for, 143
noradrenergic agents for, 188–189
risperidone for, 30, 194–195
serotonergic agents for, 189–191
serotonin-receptor antagonists for, 119
tricyclic antidepressants for, 137
Neuroleptic crisis intervention, 101
Neuroleptic malignant syndrome, 11
Neuroleptic threshold hypothesis, 94
Neuroleptics. *See also specific neuroleptics*
augmentation, with idazoxan, 141–146, **142, 144, 145**
deinstitutionalism and, 1
disadvantages of, 57
dysphoria induced by, *vs.* depression, 207–208
injectable, for noncompliant patients, 92
limitations/problems with, 153, **154**
low-potency neuroleptics, 182. *See also* Chlorpromazine
noradrenergic effects, 136–137
partial responders, 2

resistance to, 1
for schizophrenia, 106
side effects, 181. *See also* Akathisia; Akinesia
symptoms inadequately treated by, 57
treatment goals, 223
Neurotensin (NT), 67, 68
Neurotransmitter systems, 133. *See also* Noradrenergic system
Nicotine, 207
Nifedipine, 116
NMDA-PCP receptor, 75
N-methyl-D-aspartate receptor, 51
N-methyl-D-aspartate receptor antagonists, 119
N-methyl-D-aspartate-sensitive glutamate receptor, 74
NO 22-0010, **77**
Noncompliance, 92, 97
Nonresponders
augmentation algorithm for, 106–107, **107**
evaluation of, 105–106
Noradrenergic agents
clonidine, 138
development of, 51
idazoxan, 117
for negative symptoms, 188–189
neuroleptics, 136–137
propranolol, 139
tricyclic antidepressants, 137–138
Noradrenergic system
antipsychotic drug efficacy research and, 51
neurotransmission disturbances in schizophrenia, 133, 134–136
Norepinephrine
chemical structure, **134**
clozapine and, 140, 146–147
plasma levels, clozapine and, 51
in schizophrenia, 133, 135
Normetanephrine, 140
North American multicenter trial
affective symptoms and, 30–31
clinical global improvement and, 28–29
negative symptom reductions and, 195
negative symptoms and, 29–30
onset of clinical improvement and, 27–28
optimal dosage and, 26, **27–29**
positive symptoms and, 29–30, 195
risperidone side effects, 35
risperidone *vs.* haloperidol and, 31–32
NPA (N-propyl-norapomorphine), 65, **73**
NT (neurotensin), 67, 68

Obsessive-compulsive disorder, 106

Occupational impairments, negative symptoms and, 179
9-OH (9-hydroxyrisperidone), 20–21
Olanzapine
 adverse side effects, 46
 binding profile, **60**
 mechanism of action, **44,** 46, **77**
 preclinical profile, 46
 receptor blockade, broad, 59
OPC-4392, 66, **77,** 187
Opiate dependence, 122
Organic factors, *vs.* depression, 206–207
Orthostatic tachycardia, risperidone and, 35
Outcome
 long-term, negative symptomatology and, 43
 measures, 97, 98, 101. *See also* Relapse

PANSS (Positive and Negative Symptom Scale), 26, **28, 29**
Paranoia. *See* Positive symptoms
Parkinson's disease psychosis, clozapine for, 6
Partial dopamine agonists, 63–67, 187
Partial responders
 augmentation algorithm for, 106–107, **107**
 definition of, 1–2
 evaluation of, 105–106
 neurotransmitters and, 133
PCP (phencyclidine), 51, 74
PD 143188, **77**
Pemoline, 118
Pervasive developmental disorder, 106
Phencyclidine (PCP), 51, 74
Phenytoin, for clozapine-induced seizures, 11
Piribedil, 65
Platelet α_2 receptors, 135–136
Positive and Negative Symptom Scale (PANSS), 26, **28, 29**
Positive symptoms
 in acute treatment, 90, 91
 exacerbation
  anticholinergics and, 192
  L-dopa and, 185
 North American multicenter trial, 195
 psychosis. *See* Psychosis
 risperidone for, 29–30
 treatment, 108–117
  anticonvulsants for, 110–113
  antipsychotics for, 15
  benzodiazepines for, 116
  β-blockers for, 113–115
  calcium channel blockers for, 116
  clozapine for, 193, 194
  first-line augmentation agents for, 122–123
  idazoxan for, 143
  lithium for, 108–110

neuroleptics for, 153, 223
noradrenergic agents for, 117
reserpine for, 115
Posttraumatic stress disorder, 106
Postural hypotension, risperidone and, 35
(-)-3PPP. *See* Preclamol [(-)-3PPP]
Prazosin, 136–137
Preclamol [(-)-3PPP]
antidopaminergic activity, 50, 65, 66
antipsychotic efficacy, 50
dopamine receptor selectivity, **73**
mechanism of action, **77**
Prefrontal cortical dopamine system, benzodiazepines and, 156–157
Premipexole (SND 919), 65, **77**
Prodromal symptoms
targeted or intermittent treatment and, 100
vs. depression, 211
Prolactin, D_2 antagonists and, 35
Propranolol
adjunctive, 188
for akathisia, 114, 139
antipsychotic effects, 139
contraindications, 115
indications, 139
for negative symptoms, 188
for psychosis, 113–114, 139
side effects, 114–115
N-Propylnorapomorphine (NPA), 65, **73**
Psychosis
β-blockers for, 113–114
calcium channel blockers for, 116
lithium for, 108–109
rebound, 144–145
secondary negative symptoms, 181
tricyclic antidepressants and, 137
Psychosocial interventions, for depression, 215
Psychosocial stressors, 106
Psychotic exacerbations, 98, 123

Quality of life, future new antipsychotics and, 44

Raclopride, dopamine receptor selectivity, **73**
Refractory patients
augmentation treatment, 122–123
algorithm for, 106–107, **107**
evaluation of, 105–106
management of, 95–96
target symptom, 122
Refractory psychosis, *vs.* aggression, 108
Rehospitalization, 98, 101
Relapse
clozapine and, 5
dosage and, 98–99
maintenance dosages and, 97
noncompliance and, 92

Relapse *(continued)*
reasons for, 90
symptoms. *See* Prodromal symptoms
targeted or intermittent treatment and, 100
Remoxipride
binding profile, **60**
efficacy
for negative symptoms, 196–197
vs. chlorpromazine, 196
vs. haloperidol, 48–49, 196
low D_2 receptor affinity, 62–63
mechanism of action, 49, **77**
side effects, 49
Reserpine, 115
Risperidone
advantages, 61
binding profile, **60**
chemical structure, 18, **18**
clinical global improvement and, 26, **27**, 28–29
clinical studies, human, 21, 26, **22–25**
efficacy, 26–31, **27–31**
for affective symptoms, 30–31
clinical global improvement and, 28–29
for negative symptoms, 29–30, 194–195, 197
onset of clinical improvement, 27–28
optimal dosage and, 26–27, **27–31**
for positive symptoms, 29–30
extrapyramidal side effects and, 33–35
future research, 36–37
long-term studies, 36
mechanism of action, **44**, 45, **77**
metabolism, 20–21
pharmacokinetics, 20–21
preclinical and clinical studies, 45
preclinical pharmacological studies, 18, 20
receptor-binding profile, **19**, 45
serotonin receptor antagonism, 20, 119
side effects, 35–36
vs. haloperidol, 31–33, **33**
Canadian clinical trials, 32, 33, 34
Fifteen-nation trial, 30, 32–33, **33**
North American double-blind trial, 26–32, **27–32**
Ritanserin
for negative symptoms, 190
plus haloperidol, 17, 61
receptor-binding profile, **19**
serotonin blockade, 16–17

serotonin receptor antagonism, 16, 20, 119
slow-wave sleep and, 17
Roxindole, 66

SANS (Scale for the Assessment of Negative Symptoms), 143, 187, 190, 193, 194
Savoxepine, 69–70
Scale for the Assessment of Negative Symptoms (SANS), 143, 187, 190, 193, 194
SCH 39166, 61–62, **77**
Schizoaffective disorder, *vs.* depression, 211–212
Schizophrenia
acute treatment, 90–91, 93
childhood treatment-resistant, 5
chronic outpatient, 4–5
clinical psychopharmacological research, 89–90
pharmacotherapy. *See specific drugs*
symptoms. *See* Negative symptoms; Positive symptoms; *specific symptoms*
SDZ-912, **73**
SDZ DOD 647, 62
SDZ-HDC 912, 67, **77**
Sedation
clozapine-induced, 11
low-potency agents and, 182
Seizures
clozapine-induced, 11
lithium-induced, 109
Seroquel (ICI 204,636)
binding profile, 47, **60**
efficacy, 47
mechanism of action, **44**, 61, **77**
Serotonin
lithium effects on, 109
sleep and, 17
Serotonin receptor antagonists
cyproheptadine, 17
with dopamine receptor blockade, 61–62
for negative symptoms, 189–191
ritanserin. *See* Ritanserin
for schizophrenia, 16–18, 119
Serotonin receptors, clozapine and, 16
Serotonin reuptake inhibitors
adjunctive, 213
for negative symptoms, 120–121, 190
Sertindole
antipsychotic efficacy, 46
binding profile, **60**
mechanism of action, **44**, 45–46, **77**
pharmacological profile, 46
preclinical studies, 46
receptor binding profile, 61
Sigma binding site, 75–76
Simpson Neurological Rating Scale, 143, **145**
Sleep, ritanserin and, 17
Smoking, 207
SND 919 (premipexole), 65, **77**
Social impairments, negative symptoms and, 179

Stress, response,
benzodiazepines for, 155
Substance abuse, comorbid
antidipsotropic agents
and, 121, 123
cocaine, 121–122, 123
depressive-like symptoms
and, 206–207
opiate dependence,
122, 123
outcome and, 106
Substance P, 68
Suspiciousness/persecution.
See Positive symptoms

Tachycardia, clozapine-
induced, 11
Tardive dyskinesia
calcium channel blockers
for, 116
clonidine for, 138
dosage-reduction
strategies and, 96–97,
99, 101
future new antipsychotics
and, 42–43
incidence, 102
lack of, as goal for future
new antipsychotics,
42–43
neuroleptics and, 2, 57
targeted or intermittent
treatment and, 101
Targeted therapy, 99–101,
139–140
TCAs. *See* Tricyclic
antidepressants (TCAs)
TDHL, dopamine receptor
selectivity, **73**
Terguride, 66, 187
Thioridazine, **73**
Thought disorders. *See*
Positive symptoms
Tolipexole, 65
Tranylcypromine, 187
Treatment resistance, 1, 133
Treatment-responsive
patients, 42
Triazolobenzodiazepines, 161
Tricyclic antidepressants
(TCAs)
adjunctive, 213
for negative symptoms,
120
noradrenergic effects,
137–138
Trifluoperazine, **73**
Trihexyphenidyl, 191, 192

UH232, 72, **73**, **77**
United States
clozapine responder rates,
for chronic
schizophrenia, 6–7, **7**
risperidone *vs.* haloperidol
multicenter study.
See North American
multicenter trial

Valproic acid
as augmentation agent,
110, 112–113
for clozapine-induced
seizures, 11
side effects, 112–113
Verapamil, 116

Yohimbine, 136

Zacopride, 119